DEAR FUTURE EXAM SUCCESS STORY

First of all, **THANK YOU** for purchasing Mometrix study materials!

Second, congratulations! You are one of the few determined test-takers who are committed to doing whatever it takes to excel on your exam. **You have come to the right place.** We developed these study materials with one goal in mind: to deliver you the information you need in a format that's concise and easy to use.

In addition to optimizing your guide for the content of the test, we've outlined our recommended steps for breaking down the preparation process into small, attainable goals so you can make sure you stay on track.

We've also analyzed the entire test-taking process, identifying the most common pitfalls and showing how you can overcome them and be ready for any curveball the test throws you.

Standardized testing is one of the biggest obstacles on your road to success, which only increases the importance of doing well in the high-pressure, high-stakes environment of test day. Your results on this test could have a significant impact on your future, and this guide provides the information and practical advice to help you achieve your full potential on test day.

Your success is our success

We would love to hear from you! If you would like to share the story of your exam success or if you have any questions or comments in regard to our products, please contact us at **800-673-8175** or **support@mometrix.com**.

Thanks again for your business and we wish you continued success!

Sincerely,
The Mometrix Test Preparation Team

Written and edited by the Mometrix Exam Secrets Test Prep Team
Printed in the United States of America

Mometrix
TEST PREPARATION

Secrets of the

ARDMS®

Abdomen Exam Study Guide

TABLE OF CONTENTS

Introduction

Thank you for purchasing this resource! You have made the choice to prepare yourself for a test that could have a huge impact on your future, and this guide is designed to help you be fully ready for test day. Obviously, it's important to have a solid understanding of the test material, but you also need to be prepared for the unique environment and stressors of the test, so that you can perform to the best of your abilities.

For this purpose, the first section that appears in this guide is the **Secret Keys**. We've devoted countless hours to meticulously researching what works and what doesn't, and we've boiled down our findings to the five most impactful steps you can take to improve your performance on the test. We start at the beginning with study planning and move through the preparation process, all the way to the testing strategies that will help you get the most out of what you know when you're finally sitting in front of the test.

We recommend that you start preparing for your test as far in advance as possible. However, if you've bought this guide as a last-minute study resource and only have a few days before your test, we recommend that you skip over the first two Secret Keys since they address a long-term study plan.

If you struggle with **test anxiety**, we strongly encourage you to check out our recommendations for how you can overcome it. Test anxiety is a formidable foe, but it can be beaten, and we want to make sure you have the tools you need to defeat it.

Secret Key 1: Plan Big, Study Small

There's a lot riding on your performance. If you want to ace this test, you're going to need to keep your skills sharp and the material fresh in your mind. You need a plan that lets you review everything you need to know while still fitting in your schedule. We'll break this strategy down into three categories.

Information Organization

Start with the information you already have: the official test outline. From this, you can make a complete list of all the concepts you need to cover before the test. Organize these concepts into groups that can be studied together, and create a list of any related vocabulary you need to learn so you can brush up on any difficult terms. You'll want to keep this vocabulary list handy once you actually start studying since you may need to add to it along the way.

Time Management

Once you have your set of study concepts, decide how to spread them out over the time you have left before the test. Break your study plan into small, clear goals so you have a manageable task for each day and know exactly what you're doing. Then just focus on one small step at a time. When you manage your time this way, you don't need to spend hours at a time studying. Studying a small block of content for a short period each day helps you retain information better and avoid stressing over how much you have left to do. You can relax knowing that you have a plan to cover everything in time. In order for this strategy to be effective though, you have to start studying early and stick to your schedule. Avoid the exhaustion and futility that comes from last-minute cramming!

Study Environment

The environment you study in has a big impact on your learning. Studying in a coffee shop, while probably more enjoyable, is not likely to be as fruitful as studying in a quiet room. It's important to keep distractions to a minimum. You're only planning to study for a short block of time, so make the most of it. Don't pause to check your phone or get up to find a snack. It's also important to **avoid multitasking**. Research has consistently shown that multitasking will make your studying dramatically less effective. Your study area should also be comfortable and well-lit so you don't have the distraction of straining your eyes or sitting on an uncomfortable chair.

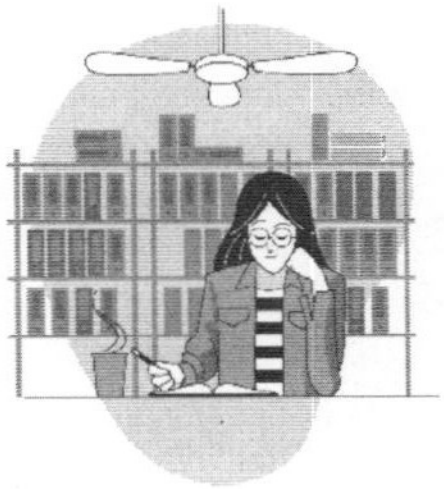

The time of day you study is also important. You want to be rested and alert. Don't wait until just before bedtime. Study when you'll be most likely to comprehend and remember. Even better, if you know what time of day your test will be, set that time aside for study. That way your brain will be used to working on that subject at that specific time and you'll have a better chance of recalling information.

Finally, it can be helpful to team up with others who are studying for the same test. Your actual studying should be done in as isolated an environment as possible, but the work of organizing the information and setting up the study plan can be divided up. In between study sessions, you can discuss with your teammates the concepts that you're all studying and quiz each other on the details. Just be sure that your teammates are as serious about the test as you are. If you find that your study time is being replaced with social time, you might need to find a new team.

Secret Key 2: Make Your Studying Count

You're devoting a lot of time and effort to preparing for this test, so you want to be absolutely certain it will pay off. This means doing more than just reading the content and hoping you can remember it on test day. It's important to make every minute of study count. There are two main areas you can focus on to make your studying count.

Retention

It doesn't matter how much time you study if you can't remember the material. You need to make sure you are retaining the concepts. To check your retention of the information you're learning, try recalling it at later times with minimal prompting. Try carrying around flashcards and glance at one or two from time to time or ask a friend who's also studying for the test to quiz you.

To enhance your retention, look for ways to put the information into practice so that you can apply it rather than simply recalling it. If you're using the information in practical ways, it will be much easier to remember. Similarly, it helps to solidify a concept in your mind if you're not only reading it to yourself but also explaining it to someone else. Ask a friend to let you teach them about a concept you're a little shaky on (or speak aloud to an imaginary audience if necessary). As you try to summarize, define, give examples, and answer your friend's questions, you'll understand the concepts better and they will stay with you longer. Finally, step back for a big picture view and ask yourself how each piece of information fits with the whole subject. When you link the different concepts together and see them working together as a whole, it's easier to remember the individual components.

Finally, practice showing your work on any multi-step problems, even if you're just studying. Writing out each step you take to solve a problem will help solidify the process in your mind, and you'll be more likely to remember it during the test.

Modality

Modality simply refers to the means or method by which you study. Choosing a study modality that fits your own individual learning style is crucial. No two people learn best in exactly the same way, so it's important to know your strengths and use them to your advantage.

For example, if you learn best by visualization, focus on visualizing a concept in your mind and draw an image or a diagram. Try color-coding your notes, illustrating them, or creating symbols that will trigger your mind to recall a learned concept. If you learn best by hearing or discussing information, find a study partner who learns the same way or read aloud to yourself. Think about how to put the information in your own words. Imagine that you are giving a lecture on the topic and record yourself so you can listen to it later.

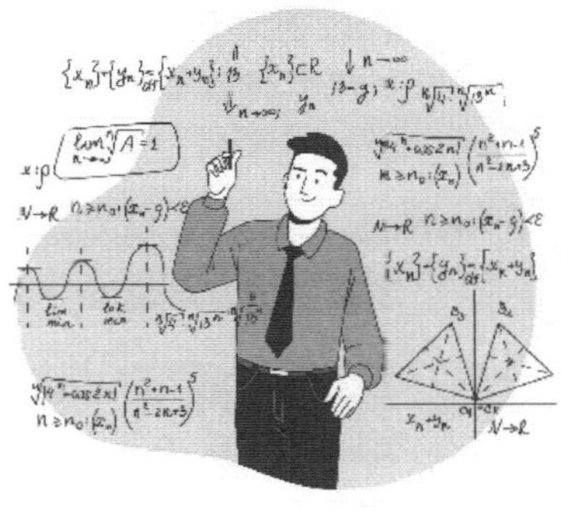

For any learning style, flashcards can be helpful. Organize the information so you can take advantage of spare moments to review. Underline key words or phrases. Use different colors for different categories. Mnemonic devices (such as creating a short list in which every item starts with the same letter) can also help with retention. Find what works best for you and use it to store the information in your mind most effectively and easily.

Secret Key 3: Practice the Right Way

Your success on test day depends not only on how many hours you put into preparing, but also on whether you prepared the right way. It's good to check along the way to see if your studying is paying off. One of the most effective ways to do this is by taking practice tests to evaluate your progress. Practice tests are useful because they show exactly where you need to improve. Every time you take a practice test, pay special attention to these three groups of questions:

- The questions you got wrong
- The questions you had to guess on, even if you guessed right
- The questions you found difficult or slow to work through

This will show you exactly what your weak areas are, and where you need to devote more study time. Ask yourself why each of these questions gave you trouble. Was it because you didn't understand the material? Was it because you didn't remember the vocabulary? Do you need more repetitions on this type of question to build speed and confidence? Dig into those questions and figure out how you can strengthen your weak areas as you go back to review the material.

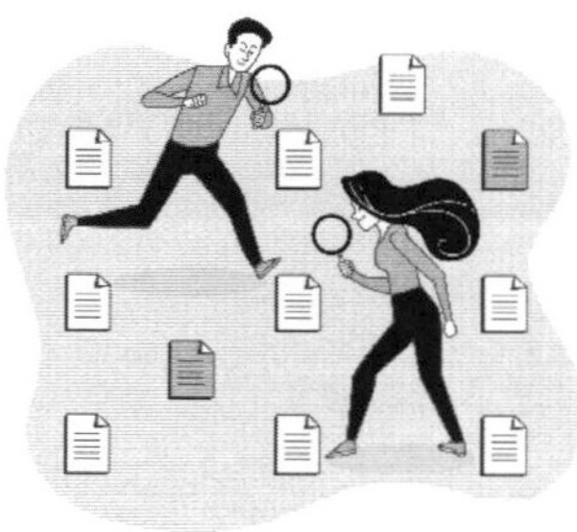

Additionally, many practice tests have a section explaining the answer choices. It can be tempting to read the explanation and think that you now have a good understanding of the concept. However, an explanation likely only covers part of the question's broader context. Even if the explanation makes perfect sense, **go back and investigate** every concept related to the question until you're positive you have a thorough understanding.

As you go along, keep in mind that the practice test is just that: practice. Memorizing these questions and answers will not be very helpful on the actual test because it is unlikely to have any of the same exact questions. If you only know the right answers to the sample questions, you won't be prepared for the real thing. **Study the concepts** until you understand them fully, and then you'll be able to answer any question that shows up on the test.

It's important to wait on the practice tests until you're ready. If you take a test on your first day of study, you may be overwhelmed by the amount of material covered and how much you need to learn. Work up to it gradually.

On test day, you'll need to be prepared for answering questions, managing your time, and using the test-taking strategies you've learned. It's a lot to balance, like a mental marathon that will have a big impact on your future. Like training for a marathon, you'll need to start slowly and work your way up. When test day arrives, you'll be ready.

Start with the strategies you've read in the first two Secret Keys—plan your course and study in the way that works best for you. If you have time, consider using multiple study resources to get different approaches to the same concepts. It can be helpful to see difficult concepts from more than one angle. Then find a good source for practice tests. Many times, the test website will suggest potential study resources or provide sample tests.

Practice Test Strategy

If you're able to find at least three practice tests, we recommend this strategy:

Untimed and Open-Book Practice

Take the first test with no time constraints and with your notes and study guide handy. Take your time and focus on applying the strategies you've learned.

Timed and Open-Book Practice

Take the second practice test open-book as well, but set a timer and practice pacing yourself to finish in time.

Timed and Closed-Book Practice

Take any other practice tests as if it were test day. Set a timer and put away your study materials. Sit at a table or desk in a quiet room, imagine yourself at the testing center, and answer questions as quickly and accurately as possible.

Keep repeating timed and closed-book tests on a regular basis until you run out of practice tests or it's time for the actual test. Your mind will be ready for the schedule and stress of test day, and you'll be able to focus on recalling the material you've learned.

Secret Key 4: Pace Yourself

Once you're fully prepared for the material on the test, your biggest challenge on test day will be managing your time. Just knowing that the clock is ticking can make you panic even if you have plenty of time left. Work on pacing yourself so you can build confidence against the time constraints of the exam. Pacing is a difficult skill to master, especially in a high-pressure environment, so **practice is vital**.

Set time expectations for your pace based on how much time is available. For example, if a section has 60 questions and the time limit is 30 minutes, you know you have to average 30 seconds or less per question in order to answer them all. Although 30 seconds is the hard limit, set 25 seconds per question as your goal, so you reserve extra time to spend on harder questions. When you budget extra time for the harder questions, you no longer have any reason to stress when those questions take longer to answer.

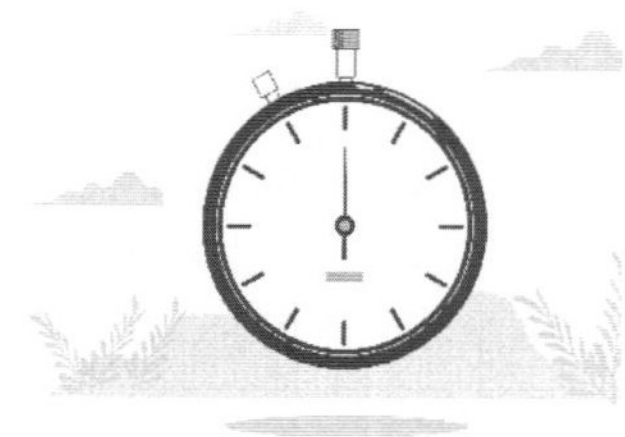

Don't let this time expectation distract you from working through the test at a calm, steady pace, but keep it in mind so you don't spend too much time on any one question. Recognize that taking extra time on one question you don't understand may keep you from answering two that you do understand later in the test. If your time limit for a question is up and you're still not sure of the answer, mark it and move on, and come back to it later if the time and the test format allow. If the testing format doesn't allow you to return to earlier questions, just make an educated guess; then put it out of your mind and move on.

On the easier questions, be careful not to rush. It may seem wise to hurry through them so you have more time for the challenging ones, but it's not worth missing one if you know the concept and just didn't take the time to read the question fully. Work efficiently but make sure you understand the question and have looked at all of the answer choices, since more than one may seem right at first.

Even if you're paying attention to the time, you may find yourself a little behind at some point. You should speed up to get back on track, but do so wisely. Don't panic; just take a few seconds less on each question until you're caught up. Don't guess without thinking, but do look through the answer choices and eliminate any you know are wrong. If you can get down to two choices, it is often worthwhile to guess from those. Once you've chosen an answer, move on and don't dwell on any that you skipped or had to hurry through. If a question was taking too long, chances are it was one of the harder ones, so you weren't as likely to get it right anyway.

On the other hand, if you find yourself getting ahead of schedule, it may be beneficial to slow down a little. The more quickly you work, the more likely you are to make a careless mistake that will affect your score. You've budgeted time for each question, so don't be afraid to spend that time. Practice an efficient but careful pace to get the most out of the time you have.

Secret Key 5: Have a Plan for Guessing

When you're taking the test, you may find yourself stuck on a question. Some of the answer choices seem better than others, but you don't see the one answer choice that is obviously correct. What do you do?

The scenario described above is very common, yet most test takers have not effectively prepared for it. Developing and practicing a plan for guessing may be one of the single most effective uses of your time as you get ready for the exam.

In developing your plan for guessing, there are three questions to address:

- When should you start the guessing process?
- How should you narrow down the choices?
- Which answer should you choose?

When to Start the Guessing Process

Unless your plan for guessing is to select C every time (which, despite its merits, is not what we recommend), you need to leave yourself enough time to apply your answer elimination strategies. Since you have a limited amount of time for each question, that means that if you're going to give yourself the best shot at guessing correctly, you have to decide quickly whether or not you will guess.

Of course, the best-case scenario is that you don't have to guess at all, so first, see if you can answer the question based on your knowledge of the subject and basic reasoning skills. Focus on the key words in the question and try to jog your memory of related topics. Give yourself a chance to bring the knowledge to mind, but once you realize that you don't have (or you can't access) the knowledge you need to answer the question, it's time to start the guessing process.

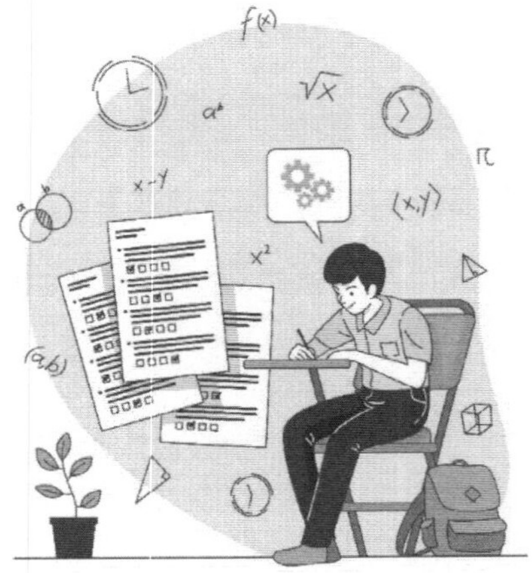

It's almost always better to start the guessing process too early than too late. It only takes a few seconds to remember something and answer the question from knowledge. Carefully eliminating wrong answer choices takes longer. Plus, going through the process of eliminating answer choices can actually help jog your memory.

Summary: Start the guessing process as soon as you decide that you can't answer the question based on your knowledge.

How to Narrow Down the Choices

The next chapter in this book (**Test-Taking Strategies**) includes a wide range of strategies for how to approach questions and how to look for answer choices to eliminate. You will definitely want to read those carefully, practice them, and figure out which ones work best for you. Here though, we're going to address a mindset rather than a particular strategy.

Your odds of guessing an answer correctly depend on how many options you are choosing from.

Number of options left	5	4	3	2	1
Odds of guessing correctly	20%	25%	33%	50%	100%

You can see from this chart just how valuable it is to be able to eliminate incorrect answers and make an educated guess, but there are two things that many test takers do that cause them to miss out on the benefits of guessing:

- Accidentally eliminating the correct answer
- Selecting an answer based on an impression

We'll look at the first one here, and the second one in the next section.

To avoid accidentally eliminating the correct answer, we recommend a thought exercise called **the $5 challenge**. In this challenge, you only eliminate an answer choice from contention if you are willing to bet $5 on it being wrong. Why $5? Five dollars is a small but not insignificant amount of money. It's an amount you could afford to lose but wouldn't want to throw away. And while losing $5 once might not hurt too much, doing it twenty times will set you back $100. In the same way, each small decision you make—eliminating a choice here, guessing on a question there—won't by itself impact your score very much, but when you put them all together, they can make a big difference. By holding each answer choice elimination decision to a higher standard, you can reduce the risk of accidentally eliminating the correct answer.

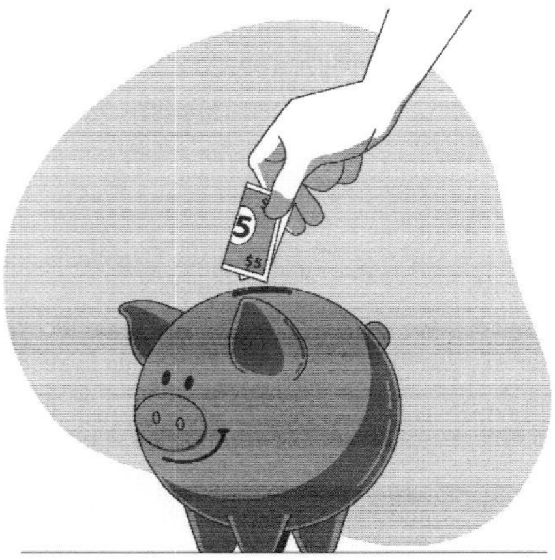

The $5 challenge can also be applied in a positive sense: If you are willing to bet $5 that an answer choice *is* correct, go ahead and mark it as correct.

Summary: Only eliminate an answer choice if you are willing to bet $5 that it is wrong.

Which Answer to Choose

You're taking the test. You've run into a hard question and decided you'll have to guess. You've eliminated all the answer choices you're willing to bet $5 on. Now you have to pick an answer. Why do we even need to talk about this? Why can't you just pick whichever one you feel like when the time comes?

The answer to these questions is that if you don't come into the test with a plan, you'll rely on your impression to select an answer choice, and if you do that, you risk falling into a trap. The test writers know that everyone who takes their test will be guessing on some of the questions, so they intentionally write wrong answer choices to seem plausible. You still have to pick an answer though, and if the wrong answer choices are designed to look right, how can you ever be sure that you're not falling for their trap? The best solution we've found to this dilemma is to take the decision out of your hands entirely. Here is the process we recommend:

Once you've eliminated any choices that you are confident (willing to bet $5) are wrong, select the first remaining choice as your answer.

Whether you choose to select the first remaining choice, the second, or the last, the important thing is that you use some preselected standard. Using this approach guarantees that you will not be enticed into selecting an answer choice that looks right, because you are not basing your decision on how the answer choices look.

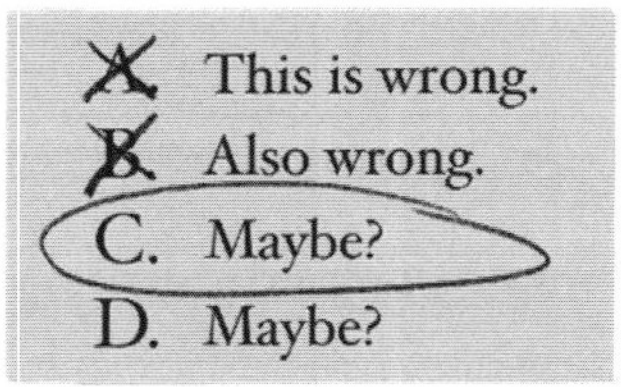

This is not meant to make you question your knowledge. Instead, it is to help you recognize the difference between your knowledge and your impressions. There's a huge difference between thinking an answer is right because of what you know, and thinking an answer is right because it looks or sounds like it should be right.

Summary: To ensure that your selection is appropriately random, make a predetermined selection from among all answer choices you have not eliminated.

Test-Taking Strategies

This section contains a list of test-taking strategies that you may find helpful as you work through the test. By taking what you know and applying logical thought, you can maximize your chances of answering any question correctly!

It is very important to realize that every question is different and every person is different: no single strategy will work on every question, and no single strategy will work for every person. That's why we've included all of them here, so you can try them out and determine which ones work best for different types of questions and which ones work best for you.

Question Strategies

⊘ Read Carefully

Read the question and the answer choices carefully. Don't miss the question because you misread the terms. You have plenty of time to read each question thoroughly and make sure you understand what is being asked. Yet a happy medium must be attained, so don't waste too much time. You must read carefully and efficiently.

⊘ Contextual Clues

Look for contextual clues. If the question includes a word you are not familiar with, look at the immediate context for some indication of what the word might mean. Contextual clues can often give you all the information you need to decipher the meaning of an unfamiliar word. Even if you can't determine the meaning, you may be able to narrow down the possibilities enough to make a solid guess at the answer to the question.

⊘ Prefixes

If you're having trouble with a word in the question or answer choices, try dissecting it. Take advantage of every clue that the word might include. Prefixes can be a huge help. Usually, they allow you to determine a basic meaning. *Pre-* means before, *post-* means after, *pro-* is positive, *de-* is negative. From prefixes, you can get an idea of the general meaning of the word and try to put it into context.

⊘ Hedge Words

Watch out for critical hedge words, such as *likely, may, can, often, almost, mostly, usually, generally, rarely,* and *sometimes*. Question writers insert these hedge phrases to cover every possibility. Often an answer choice will be wrong simply because it leaves no room for exception. Be on guard for answer choices that have definitive words such as *exactly* and *always*.

☑ Switchback Words

Stay alert for *switchbacks*. These are the words and phrases frequently used to alert you to shifts in thought. The most common switchback words are *but*, *although*, and *however*. Others include *nevertheless*, *on the other hand*, *even though*, *while*, *in spite of*, *despite*, and *regardless of*. Switchback words are important to catch because they can change the direction of the question or an answer choice.

☑ Face Value

When in doubt, use common sense. Accept the situation in the problem at face value. Don't read too much into it. These problems will not require you to make wild assumptions. If you have to go beyond creativity and warp time or space in order to have an answer choice fit the question, then you should move on and consider the other answer choices. These are normal problems rooted in reality. The applicable relationship or explanation may not be readily apparent, but it is there for you to figure out. Use your common sense to interpret anything that isn't clear.

Answer Choice Strategies

☑ Answer Selection

The most thorough way to pick an answer choice is to identify and eliminate wrong answers until only one is left, then confirm it is the correct answer. Sometimes an answer choice may immediately seem right, but be careful. The test writers will usually put more than one reasonable answer choice on each question, so take a second to read all of them and make sure that the other choices are not equally obvious. As long as you have time left, it is better to read every answer choice than to pick the first one that looks right without checking the others.

☑ Answer Choice Families

An answer choice family consists of two (in rare cases, three) answer choices that are very similar in construction and cannot all be true at the same time. If you see two answer choices that are direct opposites or parallels, one of them is usually the correct answer. For instance, if one answer choice says that quantity x increases and another either says that quantity x decreases (opposite) or says that quantity y increases (parallel), then those answer choices would fall into the same family. An answer choice that doesn't match the construction of the answer choice family is more likely to be incorrect. Most questions will not have answer choice families, but when they do appear, you should be prepared to recognize them.

☑ Eliminate Answers

Eliminate answer choices as soon as you realize they are wrong, but make sure you consider all possibilities. If you are eliminating answer choices and realize that the last one you are left with is also wrong, don't panic. Start over and consider each choice again. There may be something you missed the first time that you will realize on the second pass.

⊘ Avoid Fact Traps

Don't be distracted by an answer choice that is factually true but doesn't answer the question. You are looking for the choice that answers the question. Stay focused on what the question is asking for so you don't accidentally pick an answer that is true but incorrect. Always go back to the question and make sure the answer choice you've selected actually answers the question and is not merely a true statement.

⊘ Extreme Statements

In general, you should avoid answers that put forth extreme actions as standard practice or proclaim controversial ideas as established fact. An answer choice that states the "process should be used in certain situations, if..." is much more likely to be correct than one that states the "process should be discontinued completely." The first is a calm rational statement and doesn't even make a definitive, uncompromising stance, using a hedge word *if* to provide wiggle room, whereas the second choice is far more extreme.

⊘ Benchmark

As you read through the answer choices and you come across one that seems to answer the question well, mentally select that answer choice. This is not your final answer, but it's the one that will help you evaluate the other answer choices. The one that you selected is your benchmark or standard for judging each of the other answer choices. Every other answer choice must be compared to your benchmark. That choice is correct until proven otherwise by another answer choice beating it. If you find a better answer, then that one becomes your new benchmark. Once you've decided that no other choice answers the question as well as your benchmark, you have your final answer.

⊘ Predict the Answer

Before you even start looking at the answer choices, it is often best to try to predict the answer. When you come up with the answer on your own, it is easier to avoid distractions and traps because you will know exactly what to look for. The right answer choice is unlikely to be word-for-word what you came up with, but it should be a close match. Even if you are confident that you have the right answer, you should still take the time to read each option before moving on.

General Strategies

⊘ Tough Questions

If you are stumped on a problem or it appears too hard or too difficult, don't waste time. Move on! Remember though, if you can quickly check for obviously incorrect answer choices, your chances of guessing correctly are greatly improved. Before you completely give up, at least try to knock out a couple of possible answers. Eliminate what you can and then guess at the remaining answer choices before moving on.

⊘ Check Your Work

Since you will probably not know every term listed and the answer to every question, it is important that you get credit for the ones that you do know. Don't miss any questions through careless mistakes. If at all possible, try to take a second to look back over your answer selection and make sure you've selected the correct answer choice and haven't made a costly careless mistake (such as marking an answer choice that you didn't mean to mark). This quick double check should more than pay for itself in caught mistakes for the time it costs.

⊘ Pace Yourself

It's easy to be overwhelmed when you're looking at a page full of questions; your mind is confused and full of random thoughts, and the clock is ticking down faster than you would like. Calm down and maintain the pace that you have set for yourself. Especially as you get down to the last few minutes of the test, don't let the small numbers on the clock make you panic. As long as you are on track by monitoring your pace, you are guaranteed to have time for each question.

⊘ Don't Rush

It is very easy to make errors when you are in a hurry. Maintaining a fast pace in answering questions is pointless if it makes you miss questions that you would have gotten right otherwise. Test writers like to include distracting information and wrong answers that seem right. Taking a little extra time to avoid careless mistakes can make all the difference in your test score. Find a pace that allows you to be confident in the answers that you select.

⊘ Keep Moving

Panicking will not help you pass the test, so do your best to stay calm and keep moving. Taking deep breaths and going through the answer elimination steps you practiced can help to break through a stress barrier and keep your pace.

Final Notes

The combination of a solid foundation of content knowledge and the confidence that comes from practicing your plan for applying that knowledge is the key to maximizing your performance on test day. As your foundation of content knowledge is built up and strengthened, you'll find that the strategies included in this chapter become more and more effective in helping you quickly sift through the distractions and traps of the test to isolate the correct answer.

Now that you're preparing to move forward into the test content chapters of this book, be sure to keep your goal in mind. As you read, think about how you will be able to apply this information on the test. If you've already seen sample questions for the test and you have an idea of the question format and style, try to come up with questions of your own that you can answer based on what you're reading. This will give you valuable practice applying your knowledge in the same ways you can expect to on test day.

Good luck and good studying!

Anatomy, Perfusion, and Function

It is important for the sonographer to know the anatomy of the area being scanned in order to recognize both the normal and abnormal tissue in the patient. Understanding how the blood flows from arteries and veins throughout the circulatory system will help to identify stenosis, abnormalities in the vessels, and blood-filled organs. Some vascular structures can be seen in the mid-abdominal scan in a transverse section. Understanding locations of each organ in the abdomen will guide in imaging the area. It is important to remember that the bowel can have a different appearance depending on its contents. The small bowel is more difficult to visualize than the larger bowel, and air and gas can cause shadows on scanning and may give a mottled appearance. Bowel filled with fecal material will look distended and may be misrepresented as pathology.

Anatomy

Gallbladder and Biliary Tree

The gallbladder is about three inches long and located beneath the liver. It is shaped like a small sack. The gallbladder stores and concentrates bile (a bitter, alkaline, yellow-colored liquid that is produced by the liver and aids in the absorption and digestion of food, especially fats). The gallbladder delivers the concentrated bile to the first part of the small intestine (called the duodenum).

The gallbladder is connected to the liver and the duodenum by a series of ducts called the biliary tree. Beginning at the liver, the right hepatic duct and the left hepatic duct join to form the common hepatic duct. The gallbladder is connected to the common hepatic duct by the cystic duct to form the common bile duct. The pancreatic duct finally joins the common bile duct and the entire biliary tree ends at the duodenum (at the hepaticopancreatic ampulla or the sphincter of Oddi).

Imaging the Gallbladder

The gallbladder is an organ that is subject to image artifact during an ultrasound. It can be difficult to discern if reflectors visualized within are real. Tissue harmonics is a concept that has helped clinicians and operators gain diagnostic confidence because it tends to eliminate some signals that are not pathological. Harmonic frequencies allow the sonographer to scan patients at higher frequencies that will not only improve axial resolution but will improve the lateral resolution as well. The lateral resolution tends to improve because the wave is more narrow (higher frequency beams produce a narrower beam). Gallbladders that are imaged with harmonics have seen a decrease in improved signal-to-noise ratios, being able to see those organs that are deeper in the body, as well as eliminating reverberation artifacts. The reverberation artifacts can mimic sludge within the gallbladder.

Ultrasound operators should be aware that a high frame rate is ideal during an exam. If a sonographer would like to optimize the temporal resolution during a gallbladder exam, he or she could, of course, decrease the depth. However, if additional steps need to be taken to further improve (increase) the frame rate, the operator could decrease the field of view (the width of the sector). When the field of view is smaller, there are fewer pulses necessary to create the image, which takes less time. The frame rate (temporal resolution) is inversely proportional to the sector size of the image. A gallbladder can typically fit in a smaller sector size, especially when imaging in the transverse plane, so this is one step that can quickly be taken to improve the temporal resolution. Also, the operator should find out how many focal zones are being used. Reducing the amount of focusing may also improve temporal resolution.

Breast

The adult mammary gland forms a stalk and branches (originating at the nipple and continuing the structure to the lobules). The lobules are the functional units of the breast and are responsible for producing milk. The milk begins its passage through the breast by being expelled from the short intra-lobular terminal ducts and the longer extra-lobular terminal ducts. It then moves through the collecting ducts and finally to the nipple (through the lactiferous ducts). When the mammary gland is in the resting state, the terminal lobules (both the intra and extra) are referred to as the terminal-ductal-lobular-unit (TDLU).

Imaging the Breast

The proper transducer that will provide the most optimal imaging is a 10-15 MHz linear array depending on breast size (lower frequency for larger breasts). Proper indications for breast ultrasound include:

- Differentiation of cysts from solid masses
- Evaluation of a palpable mass that is not visible in an x-ray.
- Assessment of a mass that is not viewable in a normal mammogram (possibly due to its location)
- Evaluation of a young patient with a palpable mass

The patient should be positioned properly to conduct the examination. For example, if the patient has a right lateral breast mass, the patient should be placed in the left posterior oblique position with their right arm abducted.

Liver

General Anatomy

The liver is the largest solid organ of the body. It is also the largest gland. It weighs about three pounds in an adult and is located below the diaphragm on the right side of the abdomen. The liver is made up of four **lobes**: right, left, quadrate, and caudate lobes. The liver is secured to the diaphragm and abdominal walls by five **ligaments**. They are called the falciform (which forms a membrane-like barrier between the right and left lobes), coronary, right triangular, left triangular, and round ligaments.

The liver processes blood once it has received nutrients from the intestines via the **hepatic portal vein**. The **hepatic artery** supplies oxygen-rich blood from the abdominal aorta so that the organ can function. Blood leaves the liver through the **hepatic veins**. The liver's functional units are called **lobules** (made up of layers of liver cells). Blood enters the lobules through branches of the portal vein and hepatic artery. The blood then flows through small channels called **sinusoids**.

Fissures

The main lobar fissure definitively divides the liver into the right and left lobes. It is located along a line connecting the inferior vena cava and the gallbladder fossa. The middle hepatic vein runs within this fissure. The right segmental fissure divides the front and back parts of the right lobe of the liver. The front and back segments of the right portal vein run to the middle of each of these parts. The right hepatic vein also runs within this fissure. The left segmental fissure divides the middle and sides of the left lobe of the liver. The left intersegmental fissure delineates the top, middle, and bottom divisions of the left lobe of the liver. The ligamentum teres runs along the outer edge of the falciform ligament. The middle-third-of-left-intersegmental fissure runs along the front side of the caudate lobe.

Fossae

The left sagittal fossa is a deep groove that extends from the notch on the front of the liver to the upper border of the back. It forms a separation between the right and left lobes. The fossa for the umbilical vein provides space for the umbilical vein in the fetus. In the adult, it takes the form of the ligamentum teres (or round ligament) and is positioned between the quadrate lobe and the left lobe of the liver. The fossa for the gallbladder is a shallow "deflated balloon" shaped groove that provides space under right lobe of the liver for the gallbladder and the cystic duct. The fossa for the inferior vena cava is a short, deep cylindrical-shaped cut out that provides space for the vena cava. It extends upward and is located between the caudate lobe and the bare area of the liver.

Ultrasound Technique for the Liver

It is advisable to use the highest frequency abdominal transducer for obtaining the best image and for getting the proper penetration and depth. It is important to get the proper focal zone and depth placement for proper imaging. Take a systematic plan to view and document the liver in the transverse and longitudinal planes making sure to get the entire organ on record. Measure the longitudinal and anteroposterior diameter of the liver. Note the common hepatic duct as well as the bile duct. Color Doppler is used to identify the vasculature and record. Look for intrahepatic or extrahepatic bile ducts. Document and measure any abnormal findings including cysts, fluid in spaces, or masses.

Neck

The neck is the site of many connections from the head to the rest of the body. It includes air and food passages (trachea and esophagus), major blood vessels (including the carotid arteries and jugular veins), nerves, and the spinal cord. The neck can be divided into two distinct anatomical triangles. They are:

- The anterior triangle is made up of the front border of the sternocleidomastoid muscle, the midline of the neck, and the mandible bone.
- The posterior triangle is bordered by the back border of the sternocleidomastoid muscle, the trapezius muscles, and the clavicle bone.

The neck also contains many lymph nodes that are located within the triangles.

Salivary Glands

The salivary glands are responsible for producing saliva and releasing it into the mouth. There are three pairs of major salivary glands, they are:

- The parotid glands. These glands are located in the upper part of each cheek (near the ears). The glands release saliva at the back of the mouth (near the molars of the upper jaw).
- The submandibular glands. These glands are located in the floor of the mouth and release saliva behind the lower front teeth.
- The sublingual glands. These glands are located under the tongue and release saliva onto the floor of the mouth.

Pancreas

The pancreas is six to ten inches long and located at the back of the abdomen behind the stomach. It is a long, tapered organ. The wider (right) side is called the head and the narrower (left) side is called the tail. The head lies near the duodenum (the first part of the small intestine) and the tail ends near the spleen. The body of the pancreas lies between the head and the tail. The pancreas is made up of exocrine and endocrine tissues. The exocrine tissue secretes digestive enzymes from a series of ducts that collectively form the main pancreatic duct (that runs the length of the pancreas). The main pancreatic duct connects to the common bile duct near the duodenum. The endocrine tissue secretes hormones (such as insulin) into the bloodstream. Blood is supplied to the pancreas from the splenic artery, gastroduodenal artery, and the superior mesenteric artery.

Ultrasound Scan Technique for Pancreas Examination

The pancreas remains one of the more difficult organs to examine with ultrasound. The success of the technique depends on an accurate knowledge of the vascular structures of the pancreas and on correct adjustment of the ultrasound equipment. In preparation for examination, the patient must fast for six to eight hours. This assures that the gallbladder is dilated, the bile ducts are full, there is a minimum of bowel gas, and the stomach is empty. Real-time scanning allows the operator to view the peristalsis (contractions within the small intestine), duodenum (first part of the small intestine), and stomach. A three megahertz to five-megahertz transducer works best for adults. In children, use a five megahertz to seven and a half megahertz transducer.

The patient should be in the supine position (lying down face up). The head, neck, body, and tail of the pancreas should first be identified (in both the longitudinal and transverse plains). Next, evaluate the shape, contour, and lie of the organ. Compare the texture to that of the liver. Identify the following structures that are located in and around the pancreas:

- The superior-mesenteric artery, gastroduodenal artery, and the aorta.
- The superior-mesenteric vein, portal vein, splenic vein, left-renal vein, and the inferior-vena-cava.
- The common-bile-duct, duodenal-bulb, back wall of the stomach, and the pancreatic duct.

The left lobe of the liver, stomach and colon can be used as windows to visualize the pancreas. To achieve this, the patient needs to ingest substances (such as water, glucagon, a fatty meal, or methylcellulose) that help the ultrasound waves "pass through the window" and "see" the pancreas.

PENIS

The penis is a structure that can now be interrogated with the current advancements in ultrasound. Color Doppler has enabled clinicians to study the vascularity of this anatomical structure by minimally noninvasive means. A high-frequency transducer (longitudinal and transverse images) can demonstrate the corpus spongiosum, corpora cavernosa, and urethra, as well as the blood vessels they contain. Within the corpora cavernosa are the cavernosal arteries, which are branches of the internal pudendal artery that supply the penis with the majority of the necessary blood. Penile ultrasound is commonly performed for erectile dysfunction (ED), in which the physician will perform an injection to increase blood flow to the penis. ED may be caused when the blood vessels are unable to constrict or dilate properly to fill with blood. Blood flow velocities can be measured with ultrasound. The ultrasound technician can also check for any masses, calcifications, or fractures of the penis, or he or she can check if stones are suspected in the urethra.

URETHRA

The urethra is embedded within the corpus spongiosum (ventrally), which runs along the shaft of the penis and morphs into the head of the penis (glans penis). The corpus spongiosum is typically more echogenic when compared to the corpora cavernosa. The corpora cavernosa is paired and positioned on the dorsal and lateral surfaces of the penis and considered to be the dominant erectile tissue. They are hypoechoic on ultrasound and surrounded by a line that appears hyperechoic, which is the tunica albuginea. Together, the aforementioned structures make up the body of the penis. Ultrasound can also be used to identify the urethra and blood vessels that are present within the penis and associated measurements.

Peritoneal Cavity

Adrenal Glands

The adrenal gland is an endocrine gland that is located on the top of each kidney. It is triangular in shape and measures about one-half inch in height and three inches in length. The gland consists of a medulla (the center of the gland) and is surrounded by the cortex (the outer surface of the gland). The medulla is responsible for producing epinephrine and norepinephrine (adrenaline). The adrenal cortex produces other hormones necessary for fluid and electrolyte (salt) balance in the body (such as cortisone and aldosterone). The adrenal cortex also produces sex hormones. Using ultrasound, the adrenal gland is seen as a distinct hypoechoic structure.

Diaphragmatic Crura

The diaphragmatic crura begin as tendinous fibers forming two "legs" (crura) along the spine. The right crus "leg" is longer, larger, and more lobular. The right renal artery runs in front of the right diaphragmatic crus and in back of the inferior vena cava (IVC). The left diaphragmatic crus runs along the anterior lumbar vertebral bodies in a superior direction and inserts into the central tendon of the diaphragm. Additionally, the diaphragmatic crura of children appear large, relative to body size since crural width does not increase significantly with age.

Gastrointestinal Tract

The gastrointestinal (GI) tract begins at the mouth and continues through the esophagus, stomach, small intestine, large intestine, and rectum. Food is chewed in the mouth and travels to the stomach through the esophagus. The food is then stored and broken down in the stomach (using gastric acid produced by the stomach). The food then gradually enters the duodenum (the first part of the small intestine). The small intestine consists of three parts (the duodenum, jejunum, and the ileum). As the food travels though the small intestine, nutrients are absorbed into the bloodstream. Bile (from the liver), digestive enzymes (from the pancreas), and liquid (from the intestines) are added to assist with this process. By the time the food reaches the large intestine, most of the usable liquids and nutrients have been absorbed into the body. The resulting waste products continue to travel to the colon where they are finally eliminated from the body (through the rectum).

Layers Lining the Gut

Following are the different layers lining the gut:

- The innermost layer is called is called the mucosa. It is the moist membranous lining of the gut. It is made up of squamous cells through the esophagus, and is smooth thereafter. Connective tissue and smooth muscle are also present.
- The second layer is called the submucosa. It is made up of soft connective tissue, blood vessels, nerves and lymphatics.

- The third layer is called the muscularis-propria. It is made up of a circular inner layer, accompanied by a longitudinal outer layer consisting of smooth muscle.
- The fourth layer is called the serosa. This is a single layer that provides fluid to the gut.
- The fifth layer is called the adventitia. This is the outside connective tissue surrounding the gut.

Sonographic Technique for Imaging the Appendix

The five (or seven and a half) megahertz linear array probe should be applied with gradual and uniform pressure over the right lower quadrant. The linear array has a flat surface that makes it easier to perform compression maneuvers. The diameter of the appendix should be no larger than six millimeters. It should also be able to be compressed. A non-compressible appendix is a sign of appendicitis. If appendicitis is suspected, a five-megahertz linear array with a short focus should be utilized. If a hyperechoic focus with posterior shadowing is observed, it is a sign of an appendicolith (a calcification within the appendix).

Pelvic Ultrasound of Nonpregnant Females

The ultrasound of a nonpregnant female patient can be done in a longitudinal or transverse plane as well as the oblique plane. The uterus, including the fundus, cervix, and corpus, should be seen. The endometrium, both ovaries and fallopian tubes, and the vaginal canal should be imaged. Either transvaginal examination or transabdominal transducers can be used and an acoustic medium gel offers the best imaging medium. Measure any mass, cyst, or node imaged. Measure any uterine myomas in three dimensions and show it as intramural, submucosal, subserosal, or pedunculated. Investigate the cul-de-sac for fluid or mass. Document important laboratory tests and past medical history that may influence or support the images obtained with the ultrasound.

Prostate

The prostate is a gland of the male reproductive system. It is located in front of the rectum and just below the bladder. It is about one inch in diameter (similar to the size of a walnut) and has a cone-like shape. It is made up of two lobes called the base (located directly against the bladder) and the apex (located downward and is in contact with the superior (upper) fascia of the urogenital diaphragm). The primary purpose of the prostate is to produce fluid for semen, which then transports sperm through the urethra during the male orgasm. Blood is supplied to the prostate from the prostaticovesical arteries that branch from the internal iliac.

Capsule and Zones

The prostate is enclosed in a fibromuscular layer (stroma) that is known as the prostatic capsule. This layer is most prominent along the base of the prostate gland. Following are the zones of the prostate gland:

- Anterior Zone. The anterior zone is located in the front of the prostate gland. It is composed mostly of muscular tissue.
- Transition Zone. The transition zone is the innermost part of the prostate gland and surrounds the urethra where it passes through the organ.
- Central Zone. The central zone surrounds the transition zone.
- Peripheral Zone. The peripheral zone of the prostate gland is located in the back of the prostate gland (closest to the rectum). Prostate cancer forms in this zone eighty percent of the time.

Retroperitoneum

The retroperitoneum is simply the anatomical space behind the abdominal cavity. The following are considered retroperitoneal structures/organs:

- Kidneys
- Suprarenal Glands
- Bladder
- Ureter
- Inferior vena cava (IVC)
- Rectum
- Part of the esophagus

The following are considered secondary retroperitoneal structures/organs:

- Part of the pancreas.
- The second, third and fourth portions of the duodenum.
- The ascending and descending portions of the colon.

The borders of the retroperitoneum include the following:

- The posterior peritoneum. (front)
- The transversalis facia. (back)
- The lateral borders of the quadratus lumborum muscles and the peritoneal leaves of the mesentery. (sides)
- From the diaphragm to the pelvic brim (partitioned into the lumbar and iliac fossae). (top to bottom)

The following are spaces of the retroperitoneum:

- The posterior pararenal space and iliac fossa are located between the posterior renal fascia and the transversalis fascia. The iliac fossa is known as the "false pelvis". It contains the ureter and major branches of distal great vessels (including their lymphatics). The space merges at the bottom of the anterior pararenal space. The psoas muscle makes up the medial border. There are no organs in this space however; blood and lymph nodes (embedded in fat) are present.
- The perirenal space is surrounded by the anterior and posterior layers of the renal fascia (Gerota's fascia). This space contains the adrenal glands, kidneys, and ureters.
- The retrofascial space contains no organs and includes the posterior-abdominal-wall, muscles, nerves, lymphatics, and areolar tissue located behind the tranversalis fascia. It is divided into three compartments (psoas, lumbar and iliac).
- The anterior-pararenal space is bound in the front by posterior parietal peritoneum and in the back by the anterior renal fascia. The lateroconal fascia (the fusion of the front and back leaves of the renal fascia) forms the sides. The pancreas, duodenal sweep, ascending colon, and transverse colon lie in this space. This space merges with the bare area of the liver by the coronary ligament.

Psoas Muscles

The psoas muscles are located in the lower back. There are a total of four muscles (two psoas muscles located on each side of the spine). The larger of the two is called the psoas major. The smaller one is called the psoas minor. The psoas major originates at the spine (near the bottom of the rib cage). It then continues to the thigh bone. The psoas major functions to flex the hip. The psoas minor originates in the same area as the psoas major but continues down to the bony pelvis. It functions to flex the lower spine or lumbar area. When using ultrasound to image the retroperitoneum, the psoas muscle appears as a striated structure located in back and towards the middle of the kidney.

Scrotum

The scrotum is a part of the male anatomy that contains the testicles. It takes the form a two-sided pouch. The scrotum is separated into left and right sides by a septum (called the median raphe). Each side of the scrotum contains a testicle, an epididymis, a vas deferens, and a spermatic cord. The parietal layer of the tunica vaginalis provides an internal lining within the scrotum. The visceral layer of the tunica vaginalis surrounds the testicle except of a small bare area (located behind the testicle). The blood vessels, lymphatics, nerves, and spermatic ducts are connected to the testicle through this bare area. The scrotum has the ability to expand and contract (usually in reaction to temperature).

Epididymis

The epididymis is located on the back side of the testicle. It is made up of a head (caput), body (corpus), and tail (cauda). The head is about one quarter to one half inch wide and is also known as the globus major. A small growth may be seen on the head which is called the appendix of the epididymis. The head is located over the upper pole of the testicle. The body and tail follow the back side of the testicle to the lower pole. The efferent ducts empty into the epididymis where the spermatozoa are stored, mature, and complete the migration from the testicle to the vas deferens.

Ultrasound Appearance of the Epididymis

A complete scrotal ultrasound should include an evaluation and measurements of the testes as well as the epididymis. The epididymis consists of a head, body, and tail. The head is located posterior to the superior portion of the testis and the tail courses posterior and lateral to the inferior pole, where it evolves into the vas deferens. The ultrasound appearance of a normal epididymis tends to be coarser than the adjacent testis, but it is isoechoic to it. Epididymitis (inflammation of the epididymis) is often caused by a sexually transmitted infection or urinary tract infection, and it is a common diagnosis that can be made with ultrasound. Ultrasound evaluation of the epididymis includes bilateral interrogation with longitudinal and transverse images. Measurements of the epididymal head should be included because it will often appear edematous and hyperemic on color or power Doppler. Instead of isoechoic, the epididymis may appear hypoechoic when compared to the testis.

Seminiferous Tubules

The seminiferous tubules make up the testicular lobules (usually one to three tubules per lobule). This is the glandular part of testicles that contain the sperm producing cells. The epithelium of each tubule consists of sustentacular (or Sertoli) cells. These are tall, column-like cells that line the tubule. Located between the Sertoli cells are spermatogenic cells, which differentiate through meiosis (the cell division of reproductive or germ cells) to sperm cells. The seminiferous tubules converge to form a structure that resembles a network of tubules (called the rete testis). The rete testis then funnels the sperm cells into the efferent ducts (or vasa efferentia).

Vas Deferens

Beginning at the tail of the epididymis, the vas deferens is a narrow, muscular tube that connects the testicles to the urethra. The vas deferens is connected to the prostate and ultimately carries semen to the urethra.

Seminal Vesicles

The seminal vesicles are two sack-like glandular structures that produce part (about seventy percent) of the thick fluid (semen) that contains sperm. The thick secretions contain proteins, enzymes, fructose, mucus, vitamin C, flavins, phosphorylcholine and prostaglandins. These nutrients help the sperm cells stay alive and travel through the female reproductive system. Each vesicle is about two inches long. The vesicles are located at the base of the bladder just above and to the rear of the prostate gland.

The following ultrasound feature is present:

- The seminal vesicles appear as hypoechoic, symmetrical, irregularly shaped structures.

Testes

The testes (or testicles) are part of the male reproductive organs. The testes are glands (made up of several hundred lobules) that produce and store sperm cells used for reproduction. In addition, they serve an endocrine function by producing testosterone. Testosterone is a hormone that stimulates the production of sperm and causes male traits such as a deeper voice, larger muscles, and thick facial hair growth. They are two oval-shaped glands measuring about one inch in diameter and about one and one-half inches in length. A thick fibrous capsule called the tunica albuginea protects the testicular parenchyma. The parietal layer of the tunica vaginalis surrounds the tunica albuginea.

Spleen

The spleen is in the upper left of the abdomen. It is located behind the stomach and immediately below the diaphragm. It is about the size of a thick paperback book and weighs just over half a pound. It is made up of lymphoid tissue. The blood vessels are connected to the spleen by splenic sinuses (modified capillaries). The following peritoneal ligaments support the spleen:

- The gastrolienal ligament that connects the stomach to the spleen.
- The lienorenal ligament that connects the kidney to the spleen.
- The middle section of the phrenicocolic ligament (connects the left colic flexure to the thoracic diaphragm).

The main functions of the spleen are to filter unwanted materials from the blood (including old red blood cells) and to help fight infections. Up to ten percent of the population has one or more accessory spleens that tend to form at the hilum of the original spleen.

Superficial Structures

Sonographic Evaluation of Tendons

The proper transducer that will provide the most optimal imaging is the twelve-megahertz linear array. Tendons appear highly echogenic with a fibrillar echotexture. In comparison, normal muscles show oblique, parallel, echogenic fibers against a hypoechoic background. Proper technique is very important to avoid false hypoechogenicity due to the oblique incidence of the beam to the tendon axis.

The following ultrasound features are present in cases of tendonitis (inflammation of the tendon):

- There is a thickening of the tendon
- Echogenicity is decreased
- The margins of the tendon appear blurred
- In cases of chronic tendonitis, calcifications are present

Urinary Tract and Kidneys

The urinary tract is made up of a series of organs that produce, store, and eliminate urine. It is composed of two kidneys, two ureters, the urinary bladder, two sphincter muscles and the urethra.

The kidneys are two dark-red bean-shaped organs located at the back of the abdominal cavity just below the ribs (one on each side of the spine). Each kidney is about four inches long and two inches thick. There is an adrenal gland located above each kidney. The kidneys lie under the peritoneum in a cushion of two types of fat (perirenal and pararenal). The right kidney typically lies lower than the left due to the presence of the liver. Blood is supplied to the kidneys via two renal arteries (that branch off of the abdominal aorta). Blood leaves the kidneys through the renal veins.

Detailed anatomy of the kidneys:

- Blood is supplied to the kidneys by the renal artery. The renal artery originates from the aorta.
- The renal artery splits into three branches as it enters the kidney through the hilus. Two of these branches are located in front of the ureter and one is located behind the pelvis of the ureter.
- A total of five to six veins join together to form the renal vein. The renal vein exits the hilus directly in front of the renal artery and drains into the inferior vena cava (IVC).
- The lymph vessels run along the renal artery and join the lateral aortic lymph nodes (near the origin of the renal artery).
- Nerves line the branches of the renal vessels and begin in the renal sympathetic plexus.
- The kidneys are located within the peritoneum (retroperitoneal).
- While taking a breath, the kidneys move downward (about one inch).
- On the middle surface of each kidney lies a vertical slit called the hilus. The hilus is surrounded by a fibrous capsule and a covering of perinephric fat, then fascia.
- The following vessels and nerves are connected to the kidney at the hilus; the renal vein, the three branches of the renal artery, the ureter, the lymph vessels and sympathetic fibers.

- The expanded end of the ureter (called the pelvis) divides into two to three major calices (a calyx is a flower-shaped structure), which then divide into two to three minor calices that finally end at the renal papilla (located at the apex of a medullary pyramid).
- The kidney medulla itself consists of many pyramid-shaped funnels that empty into a central area called the renal pelvis.
- Urine is formed in the cortex to the pyramids. It is then carried by tubules to the renal pelvis where it exits the kidney through the ureter (an extension of the renal pelvis).
- The renal tubule structures are called nephrons (the functional units of the kidney). There are more than one million nephrons in the human kidney. Each nephron is about one half inch long and its walls are made up of epithelial (functional) cells.
- The nephrons are arranged in a way to filter the blood and deliver urine to the ureter for elimination from the body.

Ultrasound Technique for the Kidneys

The right kidney is best seen if the sonographer has the patient lie supine and the transducer is angled obliquely. The liver acts as the window for the sound beam. A coronal and a lateral approach are also possible. It is often helpful to have the patient roll to a right-side-up position and the transducer used at a lateral approach. To scan the left kidney, have the patient left-side up. The patient raises the arm above his head and the technician uses the coronal approach to scan through the spleen. Using the transducer at a decubitus and oblique position look for the clearest image of the left kidney with the highest frequency available. Use pillows under the patient to eliminate the cavity between the ribs and the hip bone.

When the patient is in the supine position (lying down face-up), three segments of the kidney can be observed. They are:

- A hypoechoic renal medulla zone (made up of many anechoic triangle-shaped renal pyramids).
- A renal cortex that is moderately echoic.
- A highly echoic central renal sinus.

Renal Medulla

The renal medulla shows up as hypoechoic pyramid shapes that are uniformly spaced. The pyramids are separated by linear barriers that extend to the renal sinus. The shapes are similarly sized and appear as regularly-spaced triangles. The tip of pyramid points towards the renal sinus and the base sits next to the renal cortex. The bow-shaped blood vessels are located at the base of the pyramids.

Renal Nephrons

The renal nephrons (also known as tubules) are the functional internal parts of the kidneys. Each kidney has up to five hundred thousand nephrons. Each nephron is about one half inch long. It has very thin walls made up of cells that function to filter blood and eliminate waste (in the form of urine). The nephron has one open end and one closed end. The closed end is a cup-shaped structure called Bowman's capsule. Blood (that needs to be filtered) enters Bowman's capsule and flows through a tightly wadded network of capillaries (called the glomerulus). The blood is filtered through the glomerulus and ultimately returns to the body through the renal vein. The filtrate drains towards the open end of the nephron and is further processed (for salt, water, and electrolyte balance), through the proximal convoluted tubule, Henle's loop, and the distal convoluted tubule. Any left over waste products are then eliminated from the body in the form of urine.

Bertin's Columns

Bertin's columns are "sheath-like" indentations of the kidney's outer surface (renal cortex) that penetrate the renal medulla to various depths. This is a completely normal feature of the renal cortex. Patients that have any duplication in the renal sinus show the greatest number and size of Bertin's columns. Following are the renal-mass-effect features of kidneys affected by hypertrophied Bertin's columns:

- A lateral indentation of the renal sinus.
- A clear definition from the renal sinus.
- A maximum depth that does not exceed one inch.
- The columns are contiguous with the renal cortex.
- The echogenicity resembles the renal parenchyma.
- The presence of two distinct groups of renal sinus echoes (the "split sinus" sign).
- The renal surface contour appears normal.

Urinary Bladder

The urinary bladder continuously collects urine delivered by the kidneys (via the ureters). The urinary bladder expands until it is full; the collected urine is then expelled from the body through the urethra. The urinary bladder is a hollow, muscular and elastic (bag-shaped) organ that is located on the pelvic floor. Its capacity is about eighteen ounces of urine. The stimulus to urinate (produced by the bladder's nervous receptors) is usually experienced when it is about half full. The ureters enter the bladder along the side and back of the bladder. The urethra exits the bladder from the front. The detrusor muscle (made up of smooth muscle fibers) is a layer of the urinary bladder wall. When the detrusor muscle contracts, urine is pushed from the bladder. For the urine to finally exit the bladder, both the involuntary controlled internal-sphincter and the voluntarily controlled external-sphincter must be opened.

URETER

Each ureter is about ten inches long. The ureter shows a narrowing at three different points, they are:

- Where the pelvis-of-the-ureter joins the ureter itself.
- A kinked portion that crosses the pelvic brim.
- Where the ureter penetrates the bladder wall.

The pelvis-of-the-ureter is the flower-shaped, expanded portion within the hilus of the kidney. The major calices feed into the pelvis-of-the-ureter. The ureters run downward (parallel to the spine) along the psoas muscles that also provide a measure of protection from the bones of the spine. The ureters then run along the sides of the pelvic bone and then turn forward to connect with the bladder. Blood is supplied to the ureters from the renal, testicular (or ovarian), and superior-vesical arteries.

URETHRA

The urethra connects the urinary bladder to the outside of the body. The urethra has a function to allow urine to be expelled from of the body. It also serves a reproductive function in the male, as a path for semen during ejaculation. The external-sphincter is made up of a smooth muscle that is voluntarily controlled for urination. The internal-sphincter is also made up of a smooth muscle and is controlled involuntarily (opens when the bladder is full). The urethra is about one inch long in the female and about eight inches long in the male.

Following are medical terms related to the urethra:

- Stricture: Any closure of the urethra.
- Urethritis: Inflammation of the mucous membrane located in the urethra.
- Dysuria: Difficulty in urination.
- Cystitis: Inflammation of the bladder.
- Cystostomy: Open-bladder surgery.
- Cystectomy: Surgical removal of the bladder.

Perfusion and Function

ULTRASOUND SYSTEMS THAT ENABLE VISUALIZATION OF ORGAN PERFUSION

The supply of blood to an organ is also known as organ perfusion. Ultrasound systems that have color Doppler capabilities provide users with a visual representation of blood moving through the body. The colors represent the directional flow of the red blood cells. Power Doppler can also be used, but instead of showing the direction of flow within blood vessels, it represents the presence of blood flow. Power Doppler is more sensitive than color Doppler. Some newer ultrasound systems can provide end users with an even greater ability to look at the smallest vessels — even those that display low flow velocities. This can be used when performing renal artery stenosis studies because the arteries that branch within the kidneys are quite small. These include the segmental, interlobar, arcuate, and interlobular arteries.

Bile

The functional liver cells (hepatocytes) excrete bile into the canaliculi (spaces between the liver cells). The bile drains into the right hepatic duct and the left hepatic duct that join together to form the common hepatic duct. A portion of bile travels to the gallbladder through the cystic duct. The gallbladder has a capacity to hold five tablespoons of bile. The gallbladder makes the bile ten times stronger by removing water during fasting. When a person eats a meal, the gallbladder is stimulated to contract and release the concentrated bile to the small intestine through the opening of the sphincter of Oddi (the muscle opening that controls the flow of bile and pancreatic enzymes). The liver produces about one to two liters of bile every day. Ninety five percent of the bile that enters the small intestine is recovered and returned to the liver through the terminal ileum (located at the end of the small intestine).

Bile is made up of:

- Bile Salts (cholates, chenodeoxycholate, deoxycholate): The liver produces bile salts by breaking down cholesterol. They function in a detergent-like way that breaks down dietary fats. This allows the fats to be dissolved and absorbed by the body.
- Cholesterol and Phospholipids: Four percent of bile is in the form of cholesterol. The secretion of cholesterol into bile is the major way that cholesterol is eliminated from the body. Phospholipids (a major component of cellular membranes) assist with the ability of bile salts to dissolve cholesterol.
- Bilirubin: Bilirubin is an end product of the body's metabolism of hemoglobin (the component of red blood cells that allows oxygen to be carried). This component also gives bile its characteristic yellow-green color.
- Protein: Bile proteins may play a role in regulating the intensity of bile production.

Liver

Major Functions

The liver is responsible for performing many vital functions in the body including the following:

- Production of **bile**
- Production of certain **blood plasma proteins**
- Production of **cholesterol** (and certain proteins needed to carry fats)
- Storage of excess glucose in the form of **glycogen** (that can be converted back to glucose when needed)
- Regulation of **amino acids**
- Processing of **hemoglobin** (to store iron)

- Conversion of ammonia (that is poisonous to the body) to **urea** (a waste product excreted in urine)
- **Purification** of the blood (clearing out drugs and other toxins)
- Regulation of **blood clotting**
- Controlling infections by boosting **immune factors** and removing bacteria.
- The nutrients (and drugs) that pass through the liver are converted into forms that are appropriate for the body to use.

Portal and Hepatic Veins

The portal vein drains blood from the digestive system (including the associated glands). The union of the splenic and superior mesenteric veins forms the portal vein. It divides into the left portal vein and the right portal vein before entering the liver. The left portal vein is smaller and located towards the front and top of the liver. The right portal vein is larger and located towards the back and bottom of the liver. The hepatic veins are all of the veins that carry the blood from the liver. These veins terminate into three large veins (the right hepatic vein, the middle hepatic vein, and the left hepatic vein) that open into the inferior vena cava (IVC). The right hepatic vein is the largest and joins the IVC at the right side. The middle hepatic vein joins the IVC towards the front. The left hepatic vein is the smallest and joins the IVC towards the front.

Neck

Blood Vessels

Blood is supplied to the head (through the neck) via the aortic arch. The subclavian and the common carotid arteries arise from the aortic arch. The thyrocervical trunk arises from the subclavian artery. The common carotid artery splits into two branches called the internal carotid artery and the external carotid artery. Blood is drained from the head (through the neck) via the internal and external jugular veins (the internal jugular vein is much larger than the external jugular vein). The jugular veins connect to the right subclavian vein and the brachiocephalic vein respectively.

Evaluation of Thyroid for Function and Perfusion

High-frequency ultrasound imaging of the thyroid is the best method available to evaluate the size and location of palpable masses, provide fine-needle aspiration, further assess abnormal lab values, or provide follow-up on nodules or cysts found previously. Measurements of the thyroid lobes (right and left) should be taken in the longitudinal and transverse planes to provide 3D measurements. The isthmus should also be imaged and measured. Color, power, and spectral Doppler may provide useful information pertaining to any nodules of the thyroid or any abnormalities of the neck (blood vessels or lymph nodes) and to demonstrate blood flow within the thyroid. The parathyroid may be imaged in cases of hyperparathyroidism, especially after the removal of the glands.

Peritoneal Cavity

Endocrine Functions of the Pancreas

Located amongst the groupings of exocrine cells (acini) are groups of endocrine cells (called islets of Langerhans). The islets of Langerhans are primarily made up of insulin-producing beta cells (fifty to eighty percent of the total) and glucagon-releasing alpha cells. The major hormones produced by the pancreas are insulin and glucagon. The body uses insulin to control carbohydrate metabolism by lowering the amount of sugar (glucose) in the blood. Insulin also affects fat metabolism and can change the liver's ability to release stored fat. The body also uses glucagon to control carbohydrate metabolism. Glucagon has the opposite effect of insulin in that the body uses it to increase blood sugar (glucose) levels. The levels of insulin and glucagon are balanced to maintain the optimum level of blood sugar (glucose) throughout the day.

Exocrine Functions of the Pancreas

The pancreas assists in the digestion of foods by secreting enzymes (to the small intestine) that help to break down many foods, especially fats and proteins. The precursors to these enzymes (called zymogens) are produced by groups of exocrine cells (called acini). They are converted, through a chemical reaction in the gut, to the active enzymes (such as pancreatic lipase and amylase) once they enter the small intestine. The pancreas also secretes large amounts of sodium bicarbonate to neutralize the stomach acid that reaches the small intestine. The exocrine functions of the pancreas are controlled by hormones released by the stomach and small intestine (duodenum) when food is present. The exocrine secretions of the pancreas flow into the main pancreatic duct (Wirsung's duct) and are delivered to the duodenum through the pancreatic duct.

Vascular and Ductal Landmarks

The following vascular and ductal landmarks are found on or near the pancreas:

- Portal vein and its offshoots: These are located behind the neck of pancreas at the point where the superior-mesenteric vein and the splenic vein meet.
- Splenic artery: This artery runs along the top edge of the pancreas (slightly above and behind the splenic vein).
- Common hepatic artery: This artery runs along the top of the duodenum and then splits into two branches (the proper hepatic artery and the gastroduodenal artery).
- Superior Mesenteric Artery: This artery branches off the aorta (at the lower body) and runs to the front of the duodenum and enters the small bowel's attachment to the back wall of the abdomen.
- Common Bile Duct: The common bile duct crosses in front of the portal vein and to the right of the proper hepatic artery.

Abdominal Vasculature

The arterial anatomy of the abdomen contains many major arteries including the aorta. The function of the vascular system is to transport oxygenated blood to the organs and tissue and to return the unoxygenated blood back to the lungs. The venous anatomy includes major vessels as well. Types of pathology pertaining to the abdominal vasculature have the potential to be life threatening and careful examination with ultrasound is essential. Aneurysm is the weakening of an arterial wall and rupture can be devastating. Accurate imaging and documentation of an abdominal aortic aneurysm must be monitored for growth and should not exceed two mm/year. Other arterial pathology may include arterial stenosis, arteriosclerosis, atherosclerosis, and pseudoaneurysm. Color Doppler may be used to demonstrate opposite flow directions particularly in a dissecting aneurysm.

Retroperitoneum

Evaluating Perfusion of Vessels of the Retroperitoneum

The retroperitoneum consists of the abdominal aorta, inferior vena cava (IVC), and kidneys. These structures and their associated blood vessels or branches can be assessed with gray-scale, color or power Doppler, and spectral Doppler. When evaluating the aorta, longitudinal and transverse images and measurements should be taken in the proximal (at the level of the celiac artery), mid (close to where the renal arteries branch off the aorta), and distal (proximal to the bifurcation of the iliac arteries) portions. Vessel patency may be demonstrated with the use of color and spectral Doppler as well as demonstrating any pathology including an abdominal aortic aneurysm (AAA), any atherosclerotic changes, or to observe any leaks of a postsurgical endoluminal graft. In cases of an AAA in the distal aorta, it is important to demonstrate the position of the aneurysm to the renal arteries to determine if they are also affected. The IVC can also be evaluated for the presence of a clot with gray-scale and color Doppler. The renal arteries may be evaluated for any indication of stenosis.

Visualizing as Much of the Abdominal Aorta as Possible

If the radiologist would like to visualize as much of the abdominal aorta as possible, the sonographer could use the extended field of view control on the ultrasound system. This panoramic image is available on most modern ultrasound equipment and replaces the split-screen method of demonstrating objects that are longer than the transducer face. By acquiring various volume data, the system will stitch the information together in order to display one image. This single image will offer clinicians the ability to visualize the structure at the same time. This application can be used when interrogating the abdominal aorta, and it may provide additional information regarding the exact location of aneurysms that may be encountered. Often, anatomical structures are enlarged, and it may be difficult to obtain measurements from them. These include the thyroid, testes, polycystic kidneys, musculoskeletal exams, as well as some breast lesions.

Scrotum

Blood Supply to the Scrotum

Blood is supplied to the testicles from the testicular artery which is connected to the aorta. The vas deferens and epididymis receive their blood supply from the deferential artery (a branch of the vesical artery). The peritesticular tissue receives blood from the cremasteric artery (a branch of the inferior epigastric artery). Both the deferential and cremasteric arteries are connected to the testicular artery. Blood is drained from the testicles through a network of veins originating in the mediastinum. This forms the pampiniform plexus located within the spermatic cord. The pampiniform plexus connects with three veins (the testicular, deferential, and cremasteric). The right testicular vein drains into the vena cava and the left testicular vein drains into the left renal vein.

Structures of the Scrotum and Evaluation for Perfusion

The scrotum can be evaluated sonographically to aid in the diagnosis of a multitude of symptoms the patient may experience due to trauma or infections. These include scrotal pain, swelling, mass, questionable hernia, possible torsion, varicoceles, or even to find a testis that is not palpable. The imaging technique includes documentation of the testes in the longitudinal and transverse planes with pertinent measurements. Color and spectral Doppler should also be applied, especially in cases in which torsion is a concern. The use of split-screen imaging in gray-scale and color Doppler is helpful in patients that are experiencing pain. Power Doppler may also be useful, but it should not be used without spectral interrogation. The color Doppler parameters may have to be adjusted to detect the slow flow of the testes. The spermatic cord should also be evaluated in suspected testicular torsion if possible. If a testis is not found within the scrotum, the inguinal canal must be imaged to provide further information for the clinician.

Urinary Tract and Kidneys

Functions

Following are the major functions of the kidneys and urinary tract:

- Toxin Removal: The human body is constantly accumulating toxins either from food digestion or waste products produced by cells. These toxins need to be removed quickly or they will build up to dangerous levels in the blood. The kidneys filter the toxins out of the blood and safely eliminate them for the body in the form of urine.
- Drug Removal: Many drugs are eliminated in the urine after being metabolized.
- Maintaining a proper fluid balance: The body is constantly gaining fluid (from the diet) and losing it (evaporation, urine, stool). The kidneys regulate the body's fluid balance to keep it from swelling up or becoming dehydrated.
- Electrolyte Balance: In order for cells to function properly, the concentrations of electrolytes in the blood need to be tightly controlled. The kidneys regulate this process. Here are the most important electrolytes and the organs that are sensitive to their changes:
    - Sodium – Brain and nerves
    - Potassium, Magnesium – Heart, muscle, and nerves
    - Calcium – Heart, muscle, nerves, and bone
    - Phosphorus – Muscle and bone

- Acid-Base Balance: The body's processing of proteins is sensitive to changes in acid concentration of blood. The kidneys remove excess acid to maintain the proper pH balance.
- Blood Pressure Control: The kidneys play a role in regulating blood pressure by balancing fluid and salt levels in the blood.
- Hormone Production: The kidneys produce erythropoietin (affects the bone marrow to make more red blood cells) and calcitriol (active form of vitamin D for bone health)

Renal Blood Vessels

The renal arteries are best observed when the patient is in the supine position (flat on their back) or lying on their left side (left lateral decubitus (LLD)) position. The right renal artery (RRA) and the left renal artery (LRA) originate at the aorta and run to the central renal sinus. The RRA and the LRA appear as circular tubular structures in back of the inferior vena cava (IVC). The right renal vein (RRV) and the left renal vein (LRV) run from the central renal sinus to the inferior vena cava (IVC). The renal arteries have a hypoechoic central lumen with strongly echogenic borders. The renal arteries are positioned underneath the renal veins and can be found by following their connections to the aorta. The "nutcracker" phenomenon results from compression of the left renal vein between the superior mesenteric artery and the aorta.

Pathology, Vascular Abnormalities, Trauma, and Postoperative Anatomy

Pathology

ABDOMINAL WALL

HERNIA

The abdominal wall can bulge and tear due to a natural weakness or an injury caused by strain (such as heavy lifting). This allows the lining of the abdomen to bulge through the tear and create a void. Sometimes a portion of the intestine (or other abdominal tissue) slips into this area causing pain and/or intestinal blockage. This condition is called a hernia. Most hernias occur near the groin (femoral). They sometimes occur at the navel (umbilical) or along a previous incision (ventral). Symptoms may include a physical bulge at the site of the hernia, pain during movement, or a dull ache.

Ultrasound is the modality of choice to help diagnose hernias that cannot be diagnosed clinically, especially those that tend to be small. Ultrasound is invaluable in the diagnosis of hernias because it offers a real-time visualization of the hernia contents as it protrudes through the neck. Ultrasound can be performed supine and upright, which is important because some hernias tend to reduce when the patient is lying down. The Valsalva maneuver can also be performed to increase the amount of pressure on the abdominal wall. Ultrasound can help determine if the hernia is fat containing or if the bowel is involved. Sonographers can also demonstrate reducibility of a hernia upon compression. Ultrasound machines today offers the ability to store cine clips to better demonstrate the hernia, especially during a Valsalva maneuver. Ultrasound can provide even more information such as the specific location (direct or indirect inguinal, femoral, incisional, or periumbilical hernia).

ADRENAL GLAND

Normal adrenal glands can be extremely difficult to identify in adults during an ultrasound exam. If they are visible, it is usually because they are enlarged due to a mass. Masses of the adrenal gland are often an incidental finding. An adenoma of the adrenal gland is the most likely diagnosis when a solid, hypoechoic mass is present. Metastatic disease of the adrenals is common, and this is the second most likely tumor found if a patient has a history of cancer. The normal adrenal glands may be visualized by ultrasound when performing an abdominal scan on infants, however. A neuroblastoma is a primary malignant tumor found in children that presents as a large, solid intra-abdominal mass. Adrenal hematomas may be present after trauma or vaginal delivery, and their ultrasound appearance varies with the age of the bleed. They may be anechoic early on, whereas older bleeds are more echogenic.

Pheochromocytoma

Pheochromocytoma is a tumor of the adrenal gland. These tumors cause the production of excess adrenaline into the bloodstream. Pheochromocytomas are formed in the central portion of the adrenal gland (called the adrenal medulla). The adrenal medulla is responsible for the normal production of adrenaline (that maintains blood pressure and helps the body cope with stressful situations). Pheochromocytoma can become a deadly tumor because of the severe elevation in blood pressure it causes. Symptoms may include those tied to excess adrenaline production such as sweating, headache, and a feeling of high anxiety. A serum catecholamines test (sometimes over a twenty-four-hour period) may be used to measure the level of adrenaline compounds in the blood. An abnormally high result may indicate that the condition is present.

Metastasis of the Adrenal Glands

The adrenal gland is a common site for metastases from cancers originating in the breast, lung, and kidneys. Lung cancer (due to smoking) is the leading cause of this condition. Adrenal metastasis occurs in up to ten percent of patients diagnosed with lung cancer. Most cases involve solitary, unilateral, small asymptomatic lesions. They are usually discovered incidentally when scanning the abdomen. Bilateral adrenal metastases are observed in less than three percent of patients with lung cancer. Again, most cases involve small, asymptomatic lesions. Hemorrhage (bleeding) is a rare but serious complication of adrenal metastases.

Scanning the Adrenal Glands During Pediatric Exams

The adrenal glands are part of the endocrine system and are found superior to the kidneys. The adrenal glands consist of an inner medulla and an outer cortex, and in newborns even normal adrenal glands are readily visible because higher frequency transducers can be used. The right adrenal gland can be seen more often than the left. Every pediatric abdominal ultrasound should include the adrenals to exclude any suprarenal masses such as a neuroblastoma. The adrenal glands can be difficult to visualize and require a skilled ultrasound operator, but newer ultrasound technology such as 3D, spatial compounding, and harmonic imaging have proved to be advantageous. Gray-scale is useful to determine if lesions are cystic or solid. Color and power Doppler can be used to determine if blood flow is present within any masses.

Biliary System

Disruption of the production, flow and re-circulation of bile cause most of the common symptoms of gallbladder and biliary tree disease. Patients typically develop diarrhea because the body loses the ability to digest and absorb fat (called steatorrhea). They may also develop deficiencies of the fat-soluble vitamins (Vitamin A, D, E, and K). The body may lose the ability to properly eliminate cholesterol, resulting in the elevation of blood cholesterol to dangerous levels. This increases the patient's risk for vascular diseases such as heart attack and stroke. The body may lose the ability to properly eliminate bilirubin. The bilirubin levels can then build-up, causing a yellowing of the skin and eyes (jaundice). Bile production and re-circulation is the major path for elimination of waste from the liver. Physical blockages of the gallbladder and biliary tree (caused by gallstones, injuries or tumors) may cause abnormal liver function test values, abdominal pain, and fever.

Biliary Atresia and Choledochal Cysts

Biliary atresia is a congenital blockage of the bile ducts that affects infants less than a few months old. It occurs due to the failure of the bile ducts to form normally as a fetus. Bile flow from the liver (through the biliary tree and gallbladder) is reduced or completely blocked. This can lead to liver damage (including cirrhosis of the liver) and is eventually fatal to the infant.

Choledochal cysts are congenital anomalies of the biliary tree. The common bile duct is structurally affected (the duct walls are widened and weakened), allowing bile to accumulate in the duct. The bile then forms a cyst that presses against the walls of the duct. This creates a condition in which bile may be prevented from reaching the small intestine. The bile then backs up towards the liver. The patient may experience jaundice, fever and abdominal pain (especially if the accumulated bile becomes infected).

Biliary Dyspepsia and Biliary Dyskinesia

Biliary dyspepsia is a disease in which the gastrointestinal organs, primarily the stomach and first part of the small intestine, function abnormally. It is a chronic disease in which the symptoms fluctuate in frequency and intensity. It may be caused by a lack of enough bile (to the small intestine) to process fats in the diet. The primary symptoms of dyspepsia are upper abdominal pain, belching, nausea, and abdominal bloating. The symptoms most often appear shortly after eating.

Biliary dyskinesia has symptoms of intermittent upper abdominal pain that may be accompanied by nausea and vomiting. Scarring or spasms of the sphincter of Oddi muscle may cause it. The sphincter of Oddi muscle is a small circular muscle approximately one-half inch in length. The function of this muscle is to keep the bile duct and pancreatic duct muscles closed to prevent reflux of intestinal contents into the bile duct and pancreas duct.

Biliary Obstruction to the Cystic Duct

Proximal to the Cystic Duct

Biliary obstructions proximal to the cystic duct are usually caused by carcinoma of the common bile duct (Sonographically viewed as a tubular branching of the hepatic ducts.) or metastases originating in the porta hepatis. The patient typically shows signs of jaundice and an overall itching of the body (pruritus). Alkaline phosphatase and direct bilirubin levels are also elevated. The gallbladder itself does not enlarge even after a full meal is consumed.

Distal to the Cystic Duct

Biliary obstructions distal to the cystic duct are usually caused by gallstones. Symptoms of gallstones include; upper right quadrant pain, jaundice, and itching (pruritus). Alkaline phosphatase and direct bilirubin levels are also elevated. The gallbladder itself appears small in size. The presence of gallstones appears (on the sonograph) as hyperechoic lesions along the bottom of the gallbladder. The common hepatic duct may also show the presence of gallstones.

Composition of Gallstones and Upper Normal Limits for Biliary Ducts

Ultrasound is the imaging modality of choice when a patient presents with abdominal pain (with or without jaundice) in which biliary obstruction is suspected. Biliary obstruction may be the result of cholelithiasis (gallstones), choledocholithiasis (gallstones present in the bile ducts) or masses that are compressing the bile ducts. Bile is produced in the liver, but the gallbladder is a pouch that collects bile until it is released into the small intestine to aid in digestion, such as when a fatty meal is consumed. If there is too much cholesterol (as in the majority of cases in the United States) or bilirubin in the bile, gallstones may develop. In addition to the gallbladder, the liver, bile ducts, and pancreas should also be evaluated to determine the cause of biliary obstruction. Intrahepatic ducts measuring greater than 2 mm are considered to be the cutoff normal limit. There are two hepatic ducts (right and left) that combine to form the common hepatic duct, and they typically measure less than 4 mm. The common hepatic duct merges with the cystic duct to become the common bile duct (CBD). The CBD should not measure greater than 6 mm unless the patient is elderly or has had his or her gallbladder removed.

Carcinoma of the Gallbladder

Carcinoma of the gallbladder is the most common source of carcinoma of the liver and biliary tree. Its frequency is three cases per one hundred thousand persons. It is most commonly seen in older adults (primarily women over sixty years old) with gallstones. The exact cause is unknown however it is thought to occur through years of irritation and repair cycles of the gallbladder mucosa due to gallstones. The tumor is typically made up of columnar cell adenocarcinoma.

Ultrasound features include:

- The shape of the mass is similar to the shape of the gallbladder itself.
- The echotexture is heterogeneous, solid and semi-solid.
- The gallbladder wall has been thickened.
- The adjacent liver tissue usually appears heterogeneous due to the spread of the cancer.
- The dilated biliary duct appears as a "shotgun-sign".

Cholecystitis and Cholangitis

Cholecystitis is an acute inflammation of the gallbladder. Ninety percent of the time gallstones (inside the gallbladder) cause the problem. Bile becomes trapped within the gallbladder causing irritation and pressure. Untreated, the condition may develop into a bacterial infection and ultimately perforation of the gallbladder. The primary symptom is abdominal pain (especially following a fatty meal).

Cholangitis is a condition where there is an infection present in the common bile duct. The infection commonly causes inflammation of the common bile duct resulting in symptoms of fever, chills, and pain in the right upper quadrant of the liver. It typically occurs when the common bile duct becomes clogged by a gallstone or tumor. If left untreated, serious life-threatening problems may develop (such as the spread of infection to the liver and pus-filled abscesses).

Sonographic Features and Classifications of Choledochal Cysts

Abdominal ultrasound is the preferred method for examining choledochal cysts. It does however, have limitations such as an inability to differentiate the cysts from other structures (such as the gallbladder). It may also have a decreased sensitivity due to overlying bowel gas and the presence of inflammatory diseases (such as cholangitis).

Sonographic features:

- The cyst may appear as a true cyst due to the presence of accumulated bile.
- The location of the cyst will be in the upper right quadrant of the liver region.

Choledochal cysts are put into four classifications based on their anatomy:

1. A localized widening of the common bile duct.
2. An offshoot with a pouch (connected to the common bile duct). This may resemble the cystic duct and gallbladder.
3. A widening of the common bile duct which folds into the duodenum.
4. A widening of the common bile duct plus a widening of the common hepatic duct.

Cholelithiasis and Choledocholithiasis

Cholelithiasis is the presence of gallstones within in the gallbladder (or biliary tree). Gallstones are formed when the concentrations of bile pigments and salts (both calcium and cholesterol based) become unbalanced. The gallstones themselves may very tiny or as large as one inch in diameter. In most cases, they do not cause any symptoms and are discovered incidentally. They are most likely to be found in the part of the gallbladder nearest to the opening of the cystic duct (called Hartmann's pouch).

Choledocholithiasis is the presence of gallstones in the common bile duct. About fifteen percent of patients with gallstones develop choledocholithiasis. Symptoms only occur if the flow of bile through the bile ducts becomes obstructed. This may lead to infection of the biliary tree and (if the pancreatic duct is also obstructed) pancreatitis. Typical symptoms may include pain (that worsens after a fatty meal), nausea, vomiting, fever and jaundice.

Acoustic Shadowing in Patient with Gallstones When Using a 3.5 MHz Multifrequency Probe

A sonographer can improve the resolution in what appears to be gallstones by two methods. If gallstones are suspected, but distal acoustic shadowing is not clearly identified with a 3.5 MHz probe, a sonographer can increase the frequency as high as it will go. Higher frequency transducers will create an ultrasound beam that is narrower. If the ultrasound wave is wider than the gallstone, the beam picks up signals from either side of the stone and the shadow may not be visualized as well or at all. In this case, perhaps the operator can bump the frequency all the way up to 5 MHz. Another parameter that a sonographer can adjust to create a narrow beam is to place the focal point so it is at the depth of the gallstones.

False-Positive and False-Negative Results of Ultrasound Gallstone Examination

False-positive results for a gallstone examination are possibly due to:

- Polyps within the gallbladder.
- Adenomyosis (the cells that normally line the gallbladder grow into the tissue of the gallbladder wall).
- The presence of gas in the small intestine (duodenum).
- The presence of air in the biliary tree.
- Porcelain gallbladder (calcium encrustation of the gallbladder wall).

False-negative results for a gallstone examination are possibly due to:

- The gallbladder is in its contracted state (emptied of bile).
- The cystic duct obscures the view of Hartmann's pouch (the part of the gallbladder (near the neck) where gallstones tend to collect).
- The gallstone is hidden in the fundal (bottom) cap of the gallbladder.

Cholecystectomy and Post-Surgical Function of the Biliary Tree

Cholecystectomy is the surgical removal of the gallbladder. It is most commonly performed when a patient has gallstones that are causing chronic symptoms. Each year, about five hundred thousand Americans undergo this surgery.

The major complications of this surgery are due to injury to the bile ducts. This may allow bile to leak (called a biliary fistula) into the abdominal cavity (causing a potential for infection). Also, bile duct strictures (contraction of the duct) can occur impeding the flow of bile through the biliary tree. Ultrasound examinations (before and after surgery) can help to detect complications and their source. With the gallbladder removed the sphincter of Oddi remains relaxed (loss of tonus) and the overall pressure of bile within the biliary tree drops. The flow of bile continues irrespective of fasting or eating.

Gallbladder Adenomyomatosis and Cholesterolosis

Adenomyomatosis is the most common cause of thickening of the gallbladder wall. It is caused by a benign tumor called an adenoma. It is usually without any symptoms and is discovered incidentally (through imaging or surgery). The tumor takes the form of firm, rubbery, well-defined nodule. It is located at the bottom (fundic) end of the gallbladder. It is more commonly found in women and those over thirty-five years of age. It is also a condition associated with gallstones and cholesterolosis.

Cholesterolosis (strawberry gallbladder) occurs frequently when gallstones are present. It is a chronic inflammatory condition that results in the formation of cholesterol polyps. The interior of the gallbladder appears as a strawberry. The cholesterol crystals form the background with little yellow specks of cholesterol esters making up the "seeds". The cholesterol crystals may detach from the wall of the gallbladder and form the beginning of a cholesterol stone.

Papillomas and Ultrasound Features of Benign Masses of the Gallbladder

Papilloma is a benign epithelial (made up of a layer of cells) tumor. It does not develop into cancer. There may be a single or multiple scattered tumors present.

Ultrasound features of benign tumors:

- Typically show up as small attached lumps (elevations) on the interior surface (lumen) of the gallbladder.
- Adneomyomatosis is indicated if there is reduced or no flow of bile to and from the interior of the gallbladder (through the cystic duct).
- Sometimes mistaken for a tumor (or gallstones) is a condition called Phrygian cap in which the gallbladder fundus (bottom) is abnormally tilted and a partial septum exists.

There are several other benign masses that may be observed including mucosal hyperplasia, inflammatory polyps, mucous cysts, and granulomata (caused by parasites).

Tumors in the Extrahepatic and Intrahepatic Bile Ducts

Malignant tumors that originate in the extrahepatic bile ducts (usually the common bile duct) show the same ultrasound features as pancreatic tumors. They show a distinctive pattern of the tumor bulging against a dilated common bile duct. When these tumors appear in the left and right hepatic ducts, the cancer primarily affects the ductal walls without showing signs of dilation (bulging). There is a level of difficulty in imaging these tumors since the tumor itself is not seen. The only sign is a bulging (dilation) of the duct above the tumor itself.

Malignant tumors that originate in the intrahepatic bile ducts show the same ultrasound features as primary tumors of the liver. The tumors also show a pattern of dilation to the intrahepatic ducts.

Breast

Breast Ultrasound

The breast region is a common anatomical structure that is evaluated by ultrasound. This can be performed on men or women, especially when a lump is felt to further investigate whether the mass is solid or cystic and its shape, vascularity, and borders. Breast lesions that are cystic are typically benign processes such as a cyst.

Patients often present with a lump or lumps that can be palpated with or without tenderness, nipple inversion, dimpling of the skin, or infections of the breast. Ultrasound may be performed without or in conjunction with a mammogram, depending on the patient's age and medical history or to offer guidance during a cyst aspiration or breast biopsy. In patients who are positive for breast cancer, it is common to see a hypoechoic mass that is taller than it is wide, with irregular borders and possible microcalcifications. Color Doppler and more recently, elastography, are useful methods to use when breast cancer is suspected.

Breast Masses

Breast masses are typically cystic or solid lesions. Ultrasound can distinguish between ninety-six to one hundred percent of these masses. Cystic masses have the following ultrasound features:

- The cyst will show smooth walls
- The front (anterior) and back (posterior) of the cyst will show sharply defined borders
- There will be no internal echoes
- The cyst will show posterior enhancement

Solid masses that show signs of malignancy have the following ultrasound features:

- A mass that is taller than it is wide
- Spiculation is present
- The mass shows angular margins
- The presence of a markedly hypoechoic solid lesion

Normal lymph nodes have the following ultrasound features:

- A small, ovoid structure with a hypoechoic rim and echogenic hilum.

Chest

Pleural Effusion

Pleural effusions are common in individuals with cirrhosis, lung cancer, bacterial pneumonia, and heart failure or in those that have had open heart surgery. Ultrasound can be used not only to identify the pleural effusion, but to estimate the amount of fluid present and provide real-time imaging during a thoracentesis. Ultrasound operators should evaluate suspected pleural effusions while the patient is upright using a 2–5 MHz transducer in a longitudinal plane where the diaphragm can be visualized starting just posterior to the axillary line. The operator should see the lung, diaphragm, liver or spleen, and fluid. The fluid can be assessed as either a simple or complex collection. Ultrasound can also determine whether any septa are present. Ultrasound may also be used to evaluate masses within the wall of the chest cavity. These cases are best scanned using high-frequency transducers using B-mode, color, and spectral Doppler.

Evaluating the Thymus Gland

The thymus gland can be readily evaluated with ultrasound, especially in neonates and infants due to lesser degree of ossification of their sternum and ribs. The thymus gland is part of the endocrine and lymphatic systems and is located within the mediastinum between the lungs, superior to the heart, and posterior to the sternum. The ultrasound appearance is a homogeneous, somewhat hypoechoic (when compared to the thyroid, spleen, and liver) gland with internal echogenic strands that give it a "starry sky" appearance. A normal thymus demonstrates smooth borders. Upon color Doppler interrogation, a normal thymus gland is relatively avascular. An abnormal thymus gland will have a heterogeneous, lobular appearance, often with calcifications. The size of the thymus gland varies with age as it reaches maximum size during puberty, but it is then replaced by fat and shrinks.

Chest Wall Lesions

Ultrasound can often be used as a follow-up method when a mass of the chest wall is visualized on X-rays. Radiographs may be unable to determine the various types of lesion because many of the findings are indistinguishable. Ultrasound of malignant chest masses can contribute information such as the location of the lesion, if adjacent structures are involved, if the lesion is completely solid or if it has a complex appearance, the vascularity of the lesion, and if there is a corresponding pleural effusion. Common malignant chest tumors are Ewing sarcomas and lymphomas. Benign (noncancerous) tumors that are found in the chest wall may include an abscess, lipomas, hemangiomas, and desmoid tumors. These benign processes are found more often than malignant tumors. Again, ultrasound can be used to determine the location, whether the mass is cystic or solid, the vascularity, and size.

Gastrointestinal System

Crohn's Disease

Crohn's disease causes inflammation of the gastrointestinal (GI) tract. Its exact cause is unknown; however, it may be related to an abnormal immune response by the body. It may occur in any part of the GI tract. It occurs most often in the lower part (terminal ileum) of the small intestine or colon. The inflammation and swelling can be severe enough to cause pain and repeated bouts of diarrhea. Crohn's disease is unique in that it affects all layers of the intestine. Other inflammatory intestinal diseases such as irritable bowel syndrome and ulcerative colitis only affect the top layer. Crohn's disease is also known as ileitis or enteritis. The following sonographic features may be present:

- Gut wall thickening (greater than three to five centimeters)
- Strictures
- Creeping fat (a mass effect adjacent to the bowel)
- Increasing vascularity

Adenocarcinoma of the Gastrointestinal Tract

Adenocarcinoma is the most common malignant tumor of the gastrointestinal (GI) tract. As the tumor grows, it can invade the intestinal wall. This allows the cancer to spread into adjoining lymph nodes and metastasize to other areas in the body. Most of the time adenocarcinoma occurs in the large intestine. Symptoms may include abdominal pain accompanied by nausea, bloating and loss of appetite. In advanced cases, signs of intestinal bleeding (vomiting blood and anemia) and jaundice may be present. Less than thirty five percent of patients diagnosed with adenocarcinoma of the intestines live more than five years after the cancer is discovered. This cancer is more prevalent in patients that have pre-existing Crohn's or Celiac disease.

Sonographic Indicators of Intussusception

Intussusception is often referred to as the "telescoping" of one part of the intestine within an adjacent portion, typically occurring in the region in which the small and large intestines join. This is often accompanied by inflammation and can create an obstruction. Patients often present with a right upper quadrant mass with intermittent abdominal pain, nausea, and vomiting, and often their stools will contain blood. An ultrasound of the abdomen should be performed with a high-frequency transducer, and graded compression should be used to displace any bowel gas that is present. It is important to scan the entire colon. Typical ultrasound appearances of intussusception in cross section are a target or bull's-eye appearance. A longitudinal image will often demonstrate a stacked pancake sign, and an oblique view will mimic a kidney.

Gastric Carcinoma and Lymphoma of the Stomach

Up to ninety five percent of malignant stomach tumors are carcinomas. It is the sixth leading cause of death in older males. The lesions may be fungating, ulcerated, diffuse, polypoid, or superficial. Ultrasound shows a target and may show gastric wall thickening.

Lymphoma may occur as a primary tumor of the GI tract. Up to three percent of all lymphomas are malignant stomach tumors. Symptoms may include nausea, vomiting, and weight loss. On ultrasound, the tumor appears as a large hypoechoic mass. There may be thickening of the gastric wall and a spoke-wheel pattern within the tumor.

Polyps and Leiomyomas of the Stomach

Polyps are benign tumors usually observed when the stomach is imaged full of water. The patient should be asked to drink water (immediately before the examination) to distend the stomach wall. They appear as solid masses adhering to the stomach wall. The polyps show variable echogenicity.

A leiomyoma is the most common benign tumor of the stomach. It appears as a small mass (similar to a carcinoma). It is associated with other conditions such as cholelithiasis, peptic ulcer disease, adenocarcinoma, and leiomyosarcoma. On ultrasound, it appears as a hypoechoic mass attached to the muscular layer of the stomach.

Difficulties with Scans for Abscesses

It can be difficult to determine bowels versus an abscess. The image must be done for several minutes over the worrisome area. Sometimes it helps to let the patient drink which fills the stomach and bladder with fluid. When repeating the scan over an area, make certain to duplicate the exact scan plane with every image. A water enema can also help when scanning the intestines to help differentiate a persistent bowel gas pattern from a gossypiboma. It may be necessary to rescan in a day or two to see if there is a significant change. Fat deposits also make imaging difficult and fatty areas may resemble an abscess. Ascites can be misinterpreted for an abscess but it may be helpful to place the patient in an erect or decubitus position to see if the fluid will shift. The mirror reverberations of the sound waves may show a collection of abscesses to appear as an artifact. It may help the image to scan through a different part of the bladder.

Pyloric Stenosis in Infants

Patients who have hypertrophic pyloric stenosis (HPS) will often be dehydrated, not gaining weight as expected, present with a palpable abdominal mass, and experience projectile vomiting (that does not contain bile) after being fed. HPS is the result of a thickened muscular layer of the lower third of the stomach called the pylorus. The pyloric canal allows for the passage of milk into the small intestine, but when this region is too thick, the contents are unable to continue past this point. HPS is the most common reason for surgical intervention in the first couple of months of life. Ultrasound should be performed after the baby has been fed in order to provide a dynamic study to determine if the contents are able to pass through the pyloric canal. A high-frequency transducer should be used, and the depth should be adjusted so the pylorus can be seen. With the patient supine, the pylorus can be found just posteromedial to the gallbladder and should be measured. The hypoechoic muscular layer should be less than 3 mm; an elongated pyloric canal may also be visualized, but it is a less reliable measurement (normal is less than 12 mm).

Joints

Musculoskeletal Ultrasound

Muscles appear in low to medium shades of gray with some areas of hyperechoic striations on ultrasound examination. Tendons are viewed in the longitudinal plane. Ligaments appear homogeneous and peripheral nerves look echogenic compared to ligaments and tendons. Use a high-frequency linear transducer and ensure multiple focal zones. Evaluate in two planes especially any pathology. Achilles tendon measurements are done in the transverse plane. Abdominal muscle wall exams are indicated for trauma, hernia, mass, and post-surgery patients. Musculoskeletal exams are indicated for pain, injury, inflammation, or infection. The ultrasound examination is noninvasive and done with little preparation so it can be done in an emergency setting if trauma was suspected.

Risk Factors for Developmental Dysplasia of the Hip

Developmental dysplasia of the hip (DDH) is a term used to describe a number of malformations of the hip joint. The signs of this may not always be recognized once the child is born, so this term has replaced congenital hip dysplasia. The hip is a ball-and-socket joint, but often the femoral head (ball) is not completely covered by the acetabulum (socket). Many factors play a role in this process, and it is important for the sonographer to get a thorough history from the child's caregiver, but DDH is often due to a breech position, large gestational size, oligohydramnios, or it may tend to run in families. This tends to be more prevalent in girls, especially those that are firstborn, and the left hip is impacted more often from DDH than the right side. Other clinical findings that may warrant further investigation with ultrasound for DDH include legs that are different lengths or if the folds in the thigh appear asymmetrical.

Scanning an Infant Hip for Developmental Dysplasia of the Hip

Ultrasound is often the first imaging modality chosen to help diagnose developmental dysplasia of the hip. Ultrasound can be performed in infants because the hip joint is still rather cartilaginous. The examiner should scan both hips for comparison, and this exam should not take place prior to the baby being four weeks old because the hip tends to be rather flexible (unless there is a suspected dislocation of the hip). The sonographer should document the hip in a coronal plane with the patient relaxed and in a neutral position to take any measurements. The acetabulum is best evaluated with a coronal view, and the acetabular angle can be measured. If the angle is greater than or equal to 60 degrees, this indicates a normal depth of the acetabulum. A transverse plane should be used when the hip is flexed and while performing stress views. If the femoral head changes position within the joint after light pressure is applied from a posterior approach, instability can be assumed.

Ultrasound Applications in Hip Anomalies

Ultrasound can be used in infants and children to assess when a dislocated hip is suspected or in symptoms of hip pain or when a child begins to limp. In order to diagnose a hip dislocation on ultrasound, the sonographer can perform the scan with the infant's hips flexed 90 degrees while in a transverse plane. An unstable hip is assumed when the ultrasound operator can see a difference in the relationship of the femoral head and the acetabulum when light pressure is applied from a more posterior and lateral approach. Synovitis can often be seen with ultrasound in children who are between the ages of three and eight. If the distance between the femoral neck and the external layer of the hip capsule measures more than 5 mm, then a joint effusion can be assumed. A measurement can also be taken of the contralateral side, and if the same measurements are more than 2 mm thicker on the side that is painful, a joint effusion is also diagnosed.

Liver

Sonographic Features of Cirrhosis

Cirrhosis is defined as the irreversible scarring of the liver. Scar tissue replaces healthy tissue due to the liver damage caused by toxins, viruses, and other disorders. Cirrhosis is a chronic condition that results in liver function failure and portal hypertension in its end stage. In America, cirrhosis of the liver kills about 26.000 people each year. The ability to determine the presence of cirrhosis may be difficult using ultrasound. The following features may be present:

- A coarsening of the normal liver tissue near the scarred area.
- Increased attenuation.
- Hepatosplenomegaly (an enlargement of the liver and spleen)
- Nodules on the liver's edge
- The fissures of the liver may be more visible
- Portal hypertension
- Hepatoma tumors

Congenital Liver Abnormalities

Congenital abnormalities of the liver are very rare and account for less than five percent of structural abnormalities. The possibility of a congenital abnormality should be kept in mind when an unexplained mass is encountered. One of the most well-known (of these types of abnormalities) is called Riedel's lobe. This is a triangular-shaped projection (with the base of the triangle attached to the right lobe of the liver). It is usually located towards the front of the right lobe of the liver and is more common in women than men.

Other types of congenital abnormalities of the liver include:

- Absence of one or more of its lobes
- Deformed lobes
- Decreased size of the lobes (In a normal liver, the right lobe is much larger than the left)
- Transposition of the gallbladder

Fatty Liver Disease

Non-alcoholic fatty liver (called steatosis) is a disease in which lipids accumulate to abnormally high levels in the hepatocytes. It is caused either by a physical injury to the liver or a systemic problem with the liver's ability to metabolize fat. In its milder form there is usually no damage to the liver. In its more severe form (called steatohepatitis) there is usually inflammation of the liver along with the formation of fibrous tissue. This can eventually lead to cirrhosis or liver cancer. Women are more likely to be diagnosed with fatty liver. It is found in all age groups although it is more common in middle-aged overweight/obese individuals. Contributing conditions are diabetes, high cholesterol, and high triglycerides (hyperlipidemia). The true prevalence of fatty liver is not known. The current estimate is that up to one third of American adults are affected by this disease.

Classification Grades of Liver Texture for Fatty Liver

Echogenicity increases with the amount of fatty infiltration of the liver. There is typically an enlargement of the lobe of the liver affected. The portal vein structures may be obscured because of the increased attenuation. The three grades of liver texture used to classify the degree of fatty liver are:

1. Slight increase in the fine echoes of the liver tissue with a clear, normal view of the diaphragm and blood vessel borders.
2. Moderate increase in the fine echoes of the liver tissue with a slightly blurry view of the diaphragm and blood vessel borders.
3. Heavy increase in the fine echoes of the liver tissue with poor to no ability to view the diaphragm and blood vessel borders.

Hepatocellular Disease and Bile Flow Obstruction Disease

Hepatocellular disease involves the hepatocytes (the main functional units of the liver). Since liver-function is affected by the death of liver cells, the serum liver enzyme levels will become elevated. The whole battery of liver-function-tests typically indicates the extent of disease.

Bile flow obstruction disease (cholestasis) refers to the stagnation or reduction of normal bile flow through the liver. This causes an elevation in alkaline phosphate and direct bilirubin levels in the blood. The blockage of bile can also cause problems in the livers ability to synthesize protein. This results in decreased blood albumen levels and clotting factors (PT time). The principle causes of this disease in adults are medications, cirrhosis, and a transient form that appears during pregnancy.

Liver Abscess

Abscesses of the liver are very rare (about ten cases per one hundred thousand hospitalized patients). Symptoms may include abdominal pain, diarrhea, and low fever. Typically, the white blood cell count is also elevated (called leukocytosis).

There are three major forms of liver abscess. They are:

1. Pyogenic abscess (often polymicrobial in nature). Appendicitis can cause of this type of abscess. Pyogenic abscess accounts for eighty percent of all liver abscesses.
2. Amebic abscess caused by a parasitic amoeba (entamoeba histolytica). A person contracts the parasite through the ingestion of contaminated food and water. The infection is usually confined to the colon but can spread to the liver through the portal vein.
3. Fungal abscess (most often caused by the candida species).

The following sonographic features may be present:

- The abscess may be round or oval-shaped.
- The abscess will be hyperechoic compared to the surrounding liver tissue.

Acute and Chronic Hepatitis

Hepatitis (liver inflammation) is characterized by the injury/death of liver cells and the presence of inflammatory cells in the liver tissue. Acute hepatitis generally last less than six months. Acute hepatitis can be caused by viral infections (such as mononucleosis and hepatitis virus A, B, C, D, and E), bacterial infections, amoebic infections, certain medicines, and alcohol/fungal toxins. Acute infectious viral hepatitis usually improves without any intervention. Less than 0.3 percent of patients develop liver failure in the future. Chronic hepatitis generally lasts more than six months. Chronic hepatitis can be caused by contagious viral hepatitis (such as hepatitis B, C, D), certain medicines, toxins (such as alcohol), autoimmune disease, metabolic disorders (such as Wilson's disease (retention of too much copper) and haemochromatosis (retention of too much iron). About one in five of patients with chronic hepatitis B and C are at risk of developing cirrhosis or cancer of the liver in the future.

Metastasis of the Liver

Metastasis is the process by which cancer is spread from its originating site to other areas of the body (such as the liver). Cancer cells can migrate from a primary tumor and travel (via the lymphatic and blood vessels) to affect normal, healthy tissues elsewhere in the body. The liver is a prime site for metastatic disease due the large amount of blood that travels to and through the organ. The portal vein delivers blood from the digestive tract and provides a path for colon, stomach, pancreas, biliary-tree, and intestinal cancers to spread to the liver. More than half (54%) of all liver metastases are due to colon cancer. Breast and lung cancers also frequently pass to the liver. Liver metastases usually involve an enlarged and tender liver accompanied by elevated Alk Phos, ALT and AST levels (due to the damage done to the healthy liver cells.).

Patterns of Metastases Seen in Liver Ultrasounds

Bull's eye is one type of pattern. It has an echogenic center and areas around will be a darker echopenic image. Echopenic spots appear as dark spots in the liver. Echogenic areas appear different than the surrounding liver and will appear lighter, possibly due to calcification within a mass. Cystic spots are rare and difficult to impossible to determine by ultrasound from benign cysts. Diffuse refers to numerous lesions seen throughout the liver and will raise the question of lymphoma infiltration, an immunodeficiency disease, or multi-focal hepatoma. Necrotic areas are the last pattern seen with metastases by ultrasound and these areas appear as fluid-filled centers with irregular edges. It is useful to use color and pulsed Doppler to determine where the blood flow is and if there is an obstruction or flow interruptions within the liver. It is important to remember that lower-velocity shifts noted when scanning the liver tend to indicate hemangiomas, and high-velocity shifts may be more likely to show a malignant lesion.

Hepatocellular Carcinoma

Hepatocellular Carcinoma (HCC) is a cancer that involves the normal liver cells (hepatocytes). It is somewhat rare in the United States accounting for five percent of patients with existing cirrhosis. About eighty percent of cases involving HCC occur in patients with cirrhosis of the liver. Hepatitis (B and C) infections and exposure to aflatoxins (from contaminated food) also increase a patient's risk of HCC. HCC is usually discovered during an ultrasound (or CAT) examination of the liver. Elevated blood alpha-fetoprotein (AFP) levels are also present in about seventy percent of patients with HHC. The tumor itself can be a solitary mass, have multiple nodules, or infiltrate the liver in a diffuse manner. It can affect the hepatic and portal veins, and sometimes the biliary tree. The liver usually becomes enlarged and the patient suffers from a mild fever and signs of cirrhosis.

Hepatoblastoma

Hepatoblastoma is a rare form of liver cancer that usually occurs in infancy and early childhood (the median age is one year old with most cases being diagnosed by age two). It occurs in an otherwise healthy liver. Prior hepatitis infection is not associated with the occurrence of this cancer, and it may be of genetic origin. The cancer typically appears as an abdominal mass without any symptoms. In some cases, it may be accompanied by symptoms such as weight loss, abdominal pain, loss of appetite, anemia, fever, vomiting and jaundice. The cellular structure of the tumor is epithelial or mixed (containing structural elements such as osteoid tissue). During an ultrasound examination of the tumor, the following feature is present:

- Blood flow patterns are echogenic or cystic (with internal separations).

Liver Cell Adenoma

Liver Cell Adenoma is a benign tumor made up of normal liver cells (or hepatocytes). The tumor may grow as large as twelve inches in length. This tumor occurs most commonly in young women. It is associated with oral contraceptives containing hormones. The tumor should be recognized because it can clinically mimic a hepatocellular carcinoma. The tumor may also be present in the setting of glycogen storage disorders. Since the tumor grows in the presence of hormones, it has a tendency to rupture, especially during pregnancy. During an ultrasound examination of the tumor, the following features are present:

- A solitary mass or a hyperechoic solid lesion
- The mass shows an increase in size and appears heterogeneous in the presence of tissue damage or bleeding

Focal Nodular Hyperplasia

Focal nodular hyperplasia is a rare benign tumor of the liver that takes the form of a nodule. It is composed of central scar tissue with masses of surrounding normal liver cells. The size of the nodule can vary in size and is located near the bottom edge of the liver. Typically, focal nodular hyperplasia does not cause symptoms and is normally discovered when the patient's abdomen is imaged (or during surgery). The tumor can sometimes cause pain, especially in situations where bleeding is present. The cause of focal nodular hyperplasia is uncertain. It may be caused by the abnormal development of blood vessels within the liver. Since this tumor is common in women under forty, there is a theory that this tumor is caused by hormones.

Evidence shows that the nodules enlarge in women who are on contraceptive drugs containing hormones.

Simple and Complex Liver Cysts

Simple liver cysts are also known as benign cysts, non-parasitic cysts, or solitary cysts. They occur in two to four percent of patients and are most often without any symptoms. They are typically discovered during ultrasound (or CAT) examinations of the liver. The lesion is round or oval shaped and varies in size from less than an inch to nearly eight inches. If simple cysts become symptomatic it is typically due to rupture (or bleeding) of the cyst, jaundice (due to bile obstruction), and portal hypertension.

Complex liver cysts can be caused by:

- Parasites such as echinococcus granulosus. This parasite is common among sheepherding peoples and appears as a simple oval-shaped cyst or a complex mass on a sonograph. Septations are also present.
- Hamartoma
- Hepatic cystadenoma and cystadenocarcinoma
- Cystic metastases

Other larger cysts may be due to infection caused by bacteria or infestations.

Mesenchyma Hamartoma

Mesenchymal hamartoma is a rare cystic tumor that primarily affects children under two years of age. This is the second most common benign liver tumor of childhood. It is mostly found on the right lobe of the liver. It is usually discovered through observation of an abdominal distension (caused by a non-tender mass). The tumor can be large (up to five pounds). It is made up of cysts containing clear fluid and gelatin-like material. There is some evidence that this type of tumor regresses naturally, however surgical removal is the recommended course of action.

During an ultrasound examination of the tumor, the following features are present:

- Well defined blood-flow patterns, mostly echo-free, with some web-like patterns at the border of attachment to the right lobe of the liver.

Infantile Hemangioendothelioma and Lymphoma

Infantile hemangioendothelioma is a benign tumor of the liver. There are usually multiple lesions present. The lesions are up to one inch in size and are round, smooth (with lobes) and have well defined edges. Each lesion is composed of vascular channels lined by endothelial cells. This tumor mostly affects patients who are six months of age or younger. The patients are predominantly females (by a two to one ratio). Accompanying symptoms can include gastrointestinal/internal bleeding, anemia, and jaundice. The tumor grows rapidly and then slowly regresses. The resulting liver damage may be fatal to the young patient.

A lymphoma is a rare benign slow-growing tumor made up of fatty tissue. Lymphomas are usually without any symptoms. They are typically small, but can grow up to two inches long.

Review Video: Lymphoma
Visit mometrix.com/academy and enter code: 513277

Neck

Cancers of the Neck

Neck cancers are typically squamous cell carcinomas (tumors that develop in the tissue lining the hollow organs of the body). Risk factors for cancers of the neck (and mouth) include cigarette smoking, chewing tobacco, heavy drinking, and pre-existing white patches in the mouth (called leukoplakia). The tumor types that may be seen include:

- Lymphoepithelioma
- Spindle cell carcinoma
- Verrucous cancer
- Cancers of the lymph nodes (called lymphoma)

Malignant lymph nodes show the following sonographic features:

- A rounded shape
- The echo-texture is heterogeneous
- Intranodal calcification
- Absence of an echogenic hilum

Importance of Carefully Evaluating Lymph Nodes in the Neck with Ultrasound

When a physician can palpate what is believed to be a lymph node, an ultrasound will be ordered, especially if the patient is not sick and the mass is nontender. Lymphadenopathy may be visualized incidentally when scanning other structures in the neck such as the thyroid gland. When evaluating lymph nodes, regardless of their location in the body, it is important to evaluate the shape, size, and fatty hilum of the node. Lesions in the neck that have borders that are well defined and display low-level echoes are likely lymph nodes. Ultrasound users should always apply color or power Doppler when imaging lymph nodes because a mix of peripheral and hilar (versus flow only in the hilum) flow may be an indication of a malignant node, as is a node that has lost its elliptical shape and has become more rounded.

Assessing Salivary Glands with Doppler

The salivary glands may also be scanned if an abscess, stone, cyst, or mass is suspected or if the patient has pain and swelling. Inflammatory diseases are the most prevalent reason for patients to see a clinician. Viral infections typically cause bilateral pain and swelling. A staph infection will also cause pain and swelling, and color Doppler will display hyperemia. A stone may cause obstruction of the salivary gland, and the patient may present with erythema of the affected side, especially when an abscess has formed. An abscess may not demonstrate color flow in the central portion, but rather mobile gas bubbles within a hypoechoic mass. The borders of the lesion may be difficult to identify. Salivary glands should also be scanned in the longitudinal and transverse planes with the appropriate measurements taken. Malignant lymph nodes may appear enlarged or circular, and they may have irregular borders, loss of the hilum, and peripheral blood flow visualized with color or power Doppler.

Anatomic Variants or Congenital Anomalies of the Neck

During development, the thyroid forms in the pharynx and eventually gravitates down to the base of the neck. The passageway that allows the thyroid to move will typically disappear after the thyroid is in the correct place. However, in some individuals this connection does not disappear, and, instead, it creates a pathway for cysts to materialize within. These cysts are known as thyroglossal duct cysts, and they can be seen on ultrasound located in front of the trachea in the middle of the patient's neck. They are one of the most common neck masses diagnosed in children, but they can also affect adults. Another congenital, benign cyst that may be visualized during a neck ultrasound is a branchial cleft cyst, which is in a lateral location of the neck. On ultrasound, they tend to display an anechoic or hypoechoic, ovoid appearance with thin walls. These masses tend to be compressible, and the lack of vascularity can be confirmed with color Doppler.

Evaluating the Thyroid for Masses

The thyroid gland is one of the most common superficial structures that can be evaluated with ultrasound when it is assumed that there is a mass. Often, a physician will feel an enlarged thyroid during a physical exam or the patient may have difficulty swallowing or breathing. The thyroid gland is a butterfly-shaped gland located anterior to the trachea in the inferior portion of the neck. Ultrasound can offer clinicians information such as the presence of a mass, the number and location of masses, whether the masses are cystic or solid, as well as the vascularity or demonstration of calcifications within the mass. A goiter is an enlargement of the thyroid gland, and it is the most common reason that a thyroid gland is bigger than the normal size. Other common ultrasound findings of a goiter include a heterogeneous, nodular appearance that may be difficult to penetrate well due to inflammation.

Hashimoto's Thyroiditis

Hashimoto's thyroiditis is an autoimmune disease that occurs when a person's immune system attacks the thyroid gland. When this happens, the thyroid gland becomes damaged and cannot manufacture the proper amount of thyroid-specific hormone (thyroxine) that regulates the body's metabolism (called hypothyroidism). It is more common in women than men, and is the most common cause of hypothyroidism in the United States. Symptoms may include, fatigue, depression, muscle weakness, and the presence of a goiter (swelling of the thyroid gland). The following ultrasound feature is present:

- A diffuse enlargement of the thyroid with a heterogeneous echo texture.

Grave's Disease

Grave's disease is an autoimmune disease that occurs when a person's immune system attacks the thyroid gland. When this happens, the thyroid gland becomes damaged and manufactures too much of the thyroid–specific hormone (thyroxine) that regulates the body's metabolism (called hyperthyroidism). Hyperthyroidism can increase the body's metabolism by sixty to one-hundred percent. It is more common in women than men, and is the most common cause of hyperthyroidism in the United States. Symptoms may include bulging eyeballs (Grave's ophthalmopathy), anxiety, irregular heartbeat, difficulty sleeping, weight loss, and the presence of a goiter (swelling of the thyroid gland). The following ultrasound feature is present:

- Increased vascularity of both lobes of the thyroid gland (using color Doppler)

Review Video: Graves' Disease
Visit mometrix.com/academy and enter code: 516655

Thyroid Cancer

Thyroid cancer usually begins with a nodule on the thyroid gland. Simply having a nodule on the thyroid gland is a common occurrence (especially as one ages). In most cases the nodule is benign. Symptoms may include hoarseness, neck pain, and enlarged lymph nodes. The disease typically appears in patients over thirty years old and women are affected three times more than men. The most common type of thyroid cancer is papillary or mixed (papillary and follicular). This type accounts for more than two thirds of all cases. A ten-megahertz linear array transducer will provide the most optimum scan for nodules on the thyroid gland.

Parathyroid Abnormalities

Ultrasound is a noninvasive, painless method that does not require radiation to produce images. The lower risk is also a reason why physicians will order an ultrasound first when neck masses are present or if the patient's laboratory results are abnormal. There are typically four parathyroid glands that sit on the posterior poles of the thyroid gland. Two are superior and the other two are attached to the inferior poles. Normal parathyroid glands are not often seen during an ultrasound study because of their size (3–5 mm). However, if a patient has a parathyroid adenoma, cancer, or hyperplasia (enlarged parathyroid glands), the ultrasound operator is often able to detect them. In patients that also have a multinodular goiter, it may be more difficult to penetrate the thyroid gland and parathyroid pathology may not be discerned as readily. Color or power Doppler can provide clues as to whether a mass separate from the thyroid is a lymph node or an adenoma. Parathyroid adenomas can be identified as the feeding vessels branch off of the thyroidal arteries, and they are often singular, hypoechoic, oval-shaped masses that measure less than 3 cm.

Parathyroid Adenoma

Parathyroid adenomas are benign tumors that appear on the parathyroid glands (four pea sized glands located at the front of the neck). Typically, only one of glands is affected and shows enlargement. The tumor may damage the parathyroid gland's ability to regulate the amount of calcium in the blood. This causes a condition called hyperparathyroidism (in which excess parathyroid hormone is produced). Hyperparathyroidism causes the bones to release excess calcium into the blood (resulting in hypercalcemia). The condition usually affects women over sixty years old, especially if there is a family history of the disease. Symptoms may include bone weakness, lethargy, confusion, muscle pain, kidney stones, and nausea. The following ultrasound feature is present:

- Homogeneous, hypoechoic, solid, oval-shaped nodules

Parathyroid Hyperplasia

Parathyroid hyperplasia is a disease in which all four parathyroid glands show enlargement. This enlargement is due to an increase in the number of cells making up of the parathyroid gland itself. Similar to parathyroid adenomas, hyperparathyroidism (in which excess parathyroid hormone is produced) may result. Hyperparathyroidism causes the bones to release excess calcium into the blood (resulting in hypercalcemia). Symptoms may include bone weakness, lethargy, confusion, muscle pain, kidney stones, and nausea. Parathyroid hyperplasia is responsible for about fifteen percent of all cases of hyperparathyroidism. It is more common in patients with a family history of the disease.

Carotid Body Tumor

Carotid body tumors are the most common of all the paragangliomas. Paragangliomas are tumors that arise from the paraganglion. In this case, the paraganglion is located on the outer surface (adventitia) of the carotid artery at the point where it splits (bifurcates) into the internal and external carotid arteries. It affects more women than men, and becomes more likely in patients that are fifty-years old (or older). Patients usually present with a painless neck mass that is less than one inch in diameter. Only about five to ten percent of carotid body tumors turn out to be malignant.

Pancreas

Congenital Pancreas Abnormalities

Congenital abnormalities of the pancreas are very rare. In most cases, they are related to the non-development of the organ (agenesis) or the partial development of the organ (hypoplasia). There is a condition where the head of the pancreas encircles the duodenum (called annular pancreas). Congenital cysts are the result of malformed pancreatic ducts. There is usually more than one and they can range from less than a quarter inch to up to two inches in diameter. Cystic fibrosis is a congenital abnormality that affects one in every two thousand persons. It manifests itself in problems with the liver, biliary tree, and pancreas especially as a person ages. The exocrine glands secrete an abnormal thick, sticky mucous. Eventually, cysts form due to the coagulation of the normal secretions of the liver, biliary tree and pancreas. Ultrasound shows increased echoes due to the presence of excess fibrous connective tissue.

Ultrasound Findings of Acute and Chronic Pancreatitis

Pancreatitis is inflammation of the pancreas and may be characterized as acute (sudden onset) or chronic (long term). Ultrasound is often ordered if a patient presents with epigastric or abdominal pain in the presence of elevated pancreatic enzymes. Overlying bowel gas may make it difficult to visualize the entire pancreas, but every effort should be made to see the pancreas in its entirety especially when jaundice is one of the patient's symptoms because a tumor may be the cause of obstruction. The ultrasound appearance of acute pancreatitis may demonstrate an enlarged pancreas that appears hypoechoic. Due to the inflammation, the splenic vein may not be visualized well. Chronic pancreatitis may show an enlarged gland that is more echogenic than normal. The normal pancreatic duct is less than 3 mm and is larger in the pancreatic head.

Acute Pancreatitis

Patients with acute pancreatitis may have the following symptoms:

- Moderate to severe pain in the upper abdomen (usually after a meal or heavy drinking).
- The presence of fever.

They show an increase in white cell blood count (leukocytosis) and their serum amylase and serum lipase levels rise within one to two weeks of the onset of symptoms. In adults, acute pancreatitis is typically caused by biliary tract disease or alcoholism. Up to sixty percent of patients have gallstones. Problems occur when the pancreatic juices are not allowed to flow properly due to obstructions. The pancreatic juices cause the inflammation and destruction of pancreatic tissue when they back up and migrate to the surfaces of the organ. Ultimately, equilibrium occurs as the pocketed pancreatic juices are absorbed and replenished within the pancreas. Once proper flow is restored, the acute episode of pancreatitis ends. In children, trauma, drugs, infection, or congenital anomalies typically cause acute pancreatitis.

Chronic Pancreatitis

Chronic pancreatitis consists of repeated bouts of acute pancreatitis. This results in a sustained damage and scarring of the pancreatic tissue. The healthy tissue is replaced with an atrophied, calcified and thickened fibrous tissue. Inflammation and pseudocysts are frequently present. Patients with chronic pancreatitis have attacks of abdominal pain and digestive problems. The symptoms may become more frequent as the condition worsens. The condition is usually caused by alcohol abuse; however, chronic blockage of the pancreatic duct (typically due to a narrowing of the sphincter of Oddi) is also linked to chronic pancreatitis. The following ultrasound features are present:

- There is an increase in echogenicity.
- Calcification, dilation of the pancreatic ducts, and an irregular outline are present.
- There is an enlargement of the pancreas.
- The presence of calcified stones.
- Shadowing may be present.

Hemorrhagic Pancreatitis

Patients with hemorrhagic pancreatitis may have the following symptoms:

- A decrease in hematocrit and serum calcium levels.
- Low blood pressure (hypotension) even when the patient is infused with additional blood.
- The presence of metabolic acidosis.
- The presence of adult respiratory distress syndrome.

In hemorrhagic pancreatitis, there is a sudden escape of active pancreatic enzymes that attack the pancreatic tissue (parenchyma). These enzymes break down the fat protecting the pancreas, which in turn leads to rupture of pancreatic blood vessels and bleeding. In about half of these cases the condition occurs after eating an excessively large meal or a period of very heavy drinking.

The following ultrasound features are present:

- The fresh hemorrhage appears as a well-defined single mass.
- If the hemorrhage is more than one to two weeks old it takes on cystic features.

Phlegmonous Pancreatitis and Liquefactive Necrosis

Phlegmonous pancreatitis is a condition where the intense inflammation caused by exposure to the pancreatic juices causes the pancreatic tissue to become damaged or die. The affected areas of the pancreas become hardened and thickened. The following ultrasound features are present:

- The hardened and thickened areas appear hypoechoic with good through transmission.
- There is no observation of collected pancreatic fluid.

Liquefactive necrosis (also called colliquative necrosis) is a condition where a lesion forms in an area of the pancreas that was digested by enzymes released by the pancreas during an episode of pancreatitis.

The following ultrasound features are present:

- A cystic structure is observed (without the presence of a pseudocyst).
- The cystic structure is hypoechoic.

Aneurysms Secondary to Pancreatitis and Abscess of the Pancreas

Pancreatitis can cause aneurysms of the arteries that serve the pancreas. They are mostly found on the splenic artery. They can also be found on the pancreaticdouodenal arcades including the dorsal and transverse pancreatic arteries.

An abscess of the pancreas is a collection of pus that results from pancreatic tissue death and infection. It is usually the result of pancreatitis. Its severity is related to the amount of tissue that is destroyed. It occurs in about five percent of patients that suffer from pancreatitis. There is a high probability of an abscess (in up to forty percent of patients) that suffer a bout of pancreatitis after an operation.

The following ultrasound features are present:

- A hypoechoic mass with smooth walls.
- The presence of small internal echoes.

Macrocystic Adenoma and Microcystic Adenoma

Actual pancreatic cysts (as opposed to pseudocysts) are lined by a layer of mucous and may be congenital or develop on their own. They are uncommon, accounting for less than two percent of all pancreatic tumors. Macrocystic adenoma is a slow growing, benign tumor. It usually appears as a large homogeneous cyst. It is more common in women than men. It occurs mostly on the head of the pancreas. Microcystic adenoma is a benign lesion. It consists of many small cysts lined by cells containing glycogen with little to no mucous. It is more common in women than men. It occurs mostly in the body and tail of the pancreas. The following ultrasound feature is present:

- Actual pancreatic cysts are similar in appearance to pseudocysts.

Pancreatic Pseudocysts

A pancreatic pseudocyst is a collection of pancreatic juice around the pancreas. A pseudocyst usually occurs after a bout of acute or chronic pancreatitis. The condition may appear directly (or take weeks to develop) after the patient recovers from pancreatitis. The most common location for the formation of a pseudocyst is towards the front of the pancreas at the back of the stomach. The typical symptoms may include pain in the abdomen and bloating (including digestive problems). Some complications of pseudocysts are pancreatic abscess, bleeding and blockage of the small intestine. The following ultrasound features are present:

- The presence of sharply defined smooth walls.
- Pseudocysts show usual acoustic enhancement and internal echoes.

- There may be multiple septations.
- Pseudocysts may show similarities to cystadenoma or cystadenocarcinoma.

A fluid-filled stomach, a dilated pancreatic duct, or the left renal vein varix may be mistaken for a pseudocyst.

Adenocarcinoma of the Pancreas

The majority of pancreatic cancers are adenocarcinomas. These fatal tumors occur in the pancreatic head more often than in the body or tail of the pancreas, and they affect males more often than females. These masses can be the cause of obstruction and may create symptoms such as jaundice, abdominal or back pain, and nausea and vomiting with associated weight loss. Typical ultrasound findings of an adenocarcinoma include a hypoechoic mass with irregular walls. This mass may cause enlargement of the pancreas and dilation of the pancreatic duct. Depending on the location, the adjacent vessels may be displaced either anteriorly or posteriorly, and compression of the vessels is often noted. Gray-scale and color Doppler ultrasound should be used to determine the size and vascularity of these tumors. A follow-up computed tomography or magnetic resonance imaging test will be performed if the pancreatic duct or bile ducts are dilated without sonographic visualization of a stone or mass.

Pancreatic adenocarcinoma is a fatal tumor. It is the second most common cause of death from all gastrointestinal cancers. In fact, adenocarcinoma accounts for ninety five percent of all malignant tumors originating in the pancreas. It usually affects persons sixty to eighty years old (especially males). The tumor appears in the head of the pancreas sixty to seventy percent of the time. The tumor is seldom diagnosed at an early stage. The symptoms may include jaundice, weight loss, abdominal pain, nausea/vomiting, and a general feeling of poor health/weakness. The following ultrasound features are present:

- The lesions show a different echodensity compared to the rest of the pancreas.
- The echopattern is hypoechoic.
- The borders are irregular.
- There may be an enlargement of the pancreas.
- Dilation of the pancreatic ducts is present.
- The spleen may be enlarged.
- Compression of components of the pancreatic vascular system may be caused by the tumor.

Carcinoma of the Head of the Pancreas

The term "carcinoma of the head of the pancreas" encompasses carcinoma of the sphincter-of-Oddi, the lower part of the bile duct, and the functional cells of the pancreas. It typically affects men over fifty years old. The symptoms are often weight loss followed by a progressively worsening jaundice. Back pain and overall itching (pruritus) are common. The gallbladder may be enlarged along with thrombophlebitis (inflammation with the formation of blood clots) of the splenic vein causing congestive enlargement of the spleen (splenomegaly).

The following ultrasound features are present:

- A hypoechoic mass in the pancreas.
- The superior mesenteric vessels are displaced forward.
- The presence of multiple hypoechoic nodes along the pancreas, duodenum (first part of the small intestine), and porta/superior mesenteric vessels.

Islet Cell Tumors

Islet cell tumors are derived from neuroendocrine cells. They tend to be slow growing tumors that are treatable even after they have metastasized. Islet cell tumors can produce dramatic symptoms since up to half of these tumors secrete excess hormones. There are two types of islet cell tumors. They are:

- Non-functioning islet cell tumors (ninety two percent are malignant) account for one third of all islet cell tumors. Patients with non-functioning tumors do not have any symptoms from excess hormone secretion since the tumor does not release any hormones into the blood.
- Functional islet cell tumors produce dramatic symptoms because of excess release of hormones into the blood. There are two major types of these tumors, insulinoma (a tumor that produces excessive amounts of insulin) and gastrinoma (a tumor that produces excessive amounts of gastrin).

The tumors are located mostly in the body and tail of the pancreas.

Peritoneal Cavity

Acute Appendicitis

Appendicitis is inflammation of the appendix. When the inflammation occurs suddenly, the condition is called acute appendicitis. The appendix is a small, tubular extension attached to the large intestine at the cecum. It occurs when feces, a swallowed foreign object, or a tumor obstructs the appendix. Symptoms may include a reduced appetite, nausea, vomiting, and fever. Usually, abdominal pain (located to the right of the navel) develops and becomes more severe as the condition progresses. A complication is that the appendix may rupture and cause a life-threatening infection (called infected peritonitis).

The following ultrasound features are present:

- A target lesion in the lower right quadrant.
- Thickening of the bowel wall.
- An echogenic core due to necrosis.
- The diameter of the appendix exceeds six millimeters.

Appendicitis in Pediatric Patients

When appendicitis is suspected in pediatric patients, ultrasound may be the modality of choice because it does not subject the patient to ionizing radiation. A high-frequency transducer should be used, and sonographers often ask the patient to place the probe over the region of maximum tenderness (when the patient is old enough to communicate this). Sonographic evaluation uses graded compression in order to move bowel gas out of the way and improve resolution to better visualize the appendix. The sonographer can move the transducer to the right lower quadrant to identify the ileum and cecum because the cecum is the proximal portion of the large intestine in which the appendix is located. The normal diameter of the appendix in children is 4.2 mm (6 mm in adults), and it should be compressible. Acute appendicitis will be greater than 6 mm in diameter and will not compress. Often, an inflamed appendix appears as a bull's-eye, is filled with fluid, and is hyperemic. However, an appendix that has perforated may not demonstrate blood flow. If an abscess is demonstrated, this also indicates a perforation. An appendicolith may suggest perforation, although these may be seen in patients with a normal appendix.

Ultrasound Techniques to Diagnose Pelvic Pain in Nonpregnant Women

Ultrasound on a nonpregnant woman with pelvic pain is done most successfully with the endovaginal probe. It is a safe method and essential in diagnosing the cause of pelvic pain. Ultrasound can image a torted ovary or cyst, acute pelvic inflammatory disease, and an ectopic pregnancy. The pitfalls of ultrasound for pelvic pain are that some things can still be missed, for example an abdominal pregnancy or pelvic adhesions when the uterus is impregnated. A cervical pregnancy can look like an impending abortion or a uterine fibroid can mask a pregnancy. The endovaginal transducer should be used as with other types of vaginal exams, warming the medium gel, protecting the patient's privacy, and providing patient safety while doing the scan. The patient is most often preoperatively fasting or fasting until an acute surgical condition is ruled out.

Ultrasound When Abdominal Pathology Is Suspected

An abdominal mass is usually noncompressible and does not move. With a pathological image, the bowel may show three layers giving a bull's eye appearance when cross-sectioned. Fat and connective tissue appear swollen and the texture shows an increase in echogenicity. Vasodilatations will show on color Doppler. There will be an increase in vascularity when pathology is present. Fluid, shadows, and perforations may be present on the image. In large patients a low-frequency curved linear transducer may show a clearer image and an attempt to use all techniques available must be considered to get the best image and an accurate diagnosis.

Popliteal Fossa

Baker's Cyst

A Baker's cyst is a collection of synovial fluid that builds up in a small area behind the knee. This condition is also called a popliteal cyst since it forms in the popliteal fossa. It is usually caused by injury to the knee joint such as a tear in the meniscal cartilage or degenerative arthritis. A Baker's cyst may cause symptoms such as pain, swelling, or hematoma (bruising along the back of the leg). In most cases, the condition is benign and resolves on its own. A more serious condition (such as a blood clot) may show similar characteristics and should be ruled out by techniques such as trans-illumination.

Popliteal Aneurysm

The popliteal artery is located behind the knee (in the popliteal fossa). A popliteal aneurysm occurs when this artery widens or bulges. The condition occurs most often in older adults, and may be related to atherosclerosis. Symptoms may include a pulsating lump located behind the knee, leg pain, and swelling. Since the symptoms may be similar, it is important to differentiate a popliteal aneurysm from a Baker's cyst or a blood clot in the leg veins (such as deep vein thrombosis). The presence of a popliteal aneurysm makes it more likely that other aneurysms are present in the body (such as an aortic aneurysm).

Prostate

Benign Prostatic Hyperplasia

Benign prostatic hyperplasia (BPH) is an enlargement of the prostate gland as a man ages. The prostate gland typically goes through two phases of growth. The first occurs during puberty, when the prostate typically doubles in size. Near age twenty-five, the gland begins to grow again. This second growth phase often results in BPH in older men (after age forty). More than half of men in their sixties and as many as ninety percent of men older than seventy have some symptoms of BPH. Typical symptoms include urination and bladder control problems (called prostatism) due to the enlarged prostate pressing against the urethra. The following ultrasound feature is present:

- An enlarged prostate that may be diffuse or focal.

Prostatitis

Prostatitis is the term used to describe inflammation of the prostate gland. In most cases prostatitis is caused by a bacterial infection, but it can have other causes. Symptoms include painful urination and ejaculation. Prostatitis is the most common urological disorder in men over the age of fifty however, it may occur at any age. The four major types of prostatitis are:

- Acute bacterial prostatitis is inflammation of the prostate gland caused by bacteria. Severe complications may develop if not promptly treated. This condition can be fatal if the bacterial infection is left untreated and spreads to the bloodstream.
- Chronic bacterial prostatitis is a recurrent infection and inflammation of the prostate and urinary tract. Symptoms are less severe than those associated with acute bacterial prostatitis.

- Non-bacterial prostatitis is the presence of an inflamed prostate without bacterial infection.
- Prostatodynia is the occurrence of prostatitis symptoms, without any inflammation or bacterial infection.

Malignant Tumors of the Prostate

A malignant tumor of the prostate is classified as an adenocarcinoma (or glandular cancer). It occurs when the normal semen-producing prostate cells mutate into cancer cells. It is found most often in the peripheral zone of the prostate. Eventually, the tumor may grow large enough to spread to nearby organs such as the seminal vesicles or the rectum. The tumor cells may also metastasize to the bones and bladder. Malignant tumors of the prostate occur most often in men over fifty years old. The following ultrasound features are present:

- The presence of a distinct hypoechoic lesion.
- An enlargement of the prostate.
- An irregular area of the prostate that distorts the normal hyperechoic pattern.

Ejaculatory Duct Cysts

Ejaculatory duct cysts are typically small. The cysts cause dilation of the ejaculatory duct and are most likely caused by an obstruction of the duct itself. These cysts are associated with lowered sperm counts in affected men causing infertility.

Abscess of the Prostate

An abscess should be suspected in cases where patients with acute prostatitis do not respond to treatment. Using ultrasound, abscesses of the prostate appear as an anechoic mass with or without internal echoes. Coliform bacteria (especially E-coli) cause more than seventy percent of prostatic abscesses. Surgical intervention is necessary (to drain the abscess) along with the administration of antibiotics.

Retroperitoneum

Retroperitoneal Fibrosis

Retroperitoneal fibrosis is a condition in which a large, fibrous tumor grows within the retroperitoneum. Peak incidence occurs in people aged forty to sixty, and men are affected twice as often as women. The tumor usually originates near the aorta and iliac arteries. As the tumor increases in size, it pushes against the organs that lie within the retroperitoneum. The most commonly affected organs are the kidneys and ureters. The tumor may obstruct (or even cut off) the flow of urine from the ureters to the bladder. The affected patient may complain of moderate to severe pain in the lower back (usually in the abdominal or flank areas) and difficult urination. There may also be edema (swelling) in one or both legs (due to fluid retention). Serum blood urea nitrogen (BUN) and creatinine levels may show elevation.

Lymphadenopathy

There are many lymph nodes (about six hundred) distributed throughout the human body. Palpable lymph nodes exist just under the chin (submandibular), in the arm pits (axillary) and in the groin area (inguinal). Ultrasound may be used to image lymph nodes in other areas of the body (such as the splenic-hilum, porta-hepatis, renal-hilum, and the para-aortic area). Lymphadenopathy refers to nodes that are abnormal in size (larger than one centimeter). Lymphadenopathy is categorized as "generalized" if lymph nodes are enlarged in two or more separate areas or "localized" if only one area is affected. In patients with unexplained lymphadenopathy, about three fourths of patients will present with localized lymphadenopathy and one fourth with generalized lymphadenopathy.

Scrotum

The ultrasound of the scrotum can detect carcinoma, cryptorchidism or undescended testis, and polyorchidism or the presence of more than two testes, torsion, and hernia. The ultrasound should find a small amount of fluid in the scrotal sac surrounding each testis and the vascular structures known to be present. Care should be taken to protect the privacy of the patient when performing the scrotal ultrasound. The testis should measure 4 cm in length and 2 cm in height and 3 cm in width in an adult male patient. If the measurements are far from the normal expected, suspicion of testicular carcinoma should be considered. Use the highest frequency linear transducer to obtain the best depth and clear image. Place the penis on the lower abdomen and cover with a towel for privacy. Evaluate the scrotum from the superior to the inferior walls and medial to lateral in both sagittal and transverse planes. Use a transabdominal or endorectal transducer for the prostate examination.

Scrotal Hernia and Hematoma of the Testicle

A scrotal hernia occurs when a section of the bowel bulges into the scrotum. The affected patient usually presents with an enlarged scrotum. The following ultrasound feature is present:

- Peristalsing loops of the bowel are observed in the scrotum.

Trauma to the testicle may cause injury and bleeding. The following ultrasound features are present:

- The normal homogeneous appearance of the testicle may be altered.
- Hematomas of the epididymis or scrotal wall will have variable appearances.
- The age of the hematoma affects the observed features.
- At first, the hematoma will appear hypoechoic.
- As the hematoma ages, the appearance becomes more echogenic.

Epididymitis

Epididymitis is an infection of the epididymis that eventually spreads to the testicle. The scrotum typically becomes swollen and tender. In most cases, the infection occurs on one side of the scrotum. Patients usually present with fever and painful urination. The following ultrasound features are present:

- The head of the epididymis shows enlargement (with decreased echogenicity in the swollen area).
- A reactive hydrocele (an accumulation of anechoic fluid in the scrotum surrounding the testicle and epididymis) may be present.
- Color Doppler shows an increased amount of blood flow in the affected epididymis.
- In the event an abscess has formed, complex cystic structures may be observed.

Role of Ultrasound in Cases of Cryptorchidism

Cryptorchidism can be defined as the failure of one or both testes to descend into the scrotum. If a clinician suspects an undescended testis and cannot palpate it within the inguinal canal, an ultrasound exam will often be ordered because it does not use ionizing radiation. When an ultrasound exam is ordered, it is important to perform a full scrotal ultrasound to confirm that the scrotum does not contain one or both testes. The gray-scale images should include a side-by-side comparison so that the radiologist can clearly see the missing testis. Once the measurements, color, and spectral Doppler images have been documented, the sonographer should scan the inguinal canal on the side of the missing testis. If located, measurements and color Doppler images should be provided. If the testis is not found in the inguinal canal, it is important to remember that testes form in the abdomen and may be found as superiorly as the kidneys. If it cannot be located, it may be beneficial to have a clinician present during the scan.

Evaluating Parenchymal Diseases of the Testes

When a patient presents with a palpable scrotal mass, swelling, or pain, he will be sent to the ultrasound laboratory for evaluation. Intratesticular neoplasms tend to be malignant, whereas extratesticular masses tend to be associated with a benign process. Intratesticular lesions can be easily identified with ultrasound, and these can include primary or metastatic tumors. Primary lesions will typically look like a hypoechoic, hyperemic mass with borders that are clearly defined. This mass may display cystic components as well. Microlithiasis is frequently diagnosed by ultrasound and appears as multiple echogenic foci within the testes. Orchitis will demonstrate as an enlarged testicle with a heterogeneous appearance. It is helpful for diagnosis to determine if a patient has elevated labs, fever, or chills because orchitis is an infection that has spread, but it may look similar to a malignant tumor.

Ectasia of the Rete Testis

During a testicular ultrasound, a thin echogenic line may be visualized in the middle (hilum) of the testes. This line is the mediastinum testis, which is a continuation of the tunica albuginea (the fibrous capsule that encases the testes) and contains blood vessels, nerves, and seminiferous tubules. The rete testis is a region in which the various tubules join together to propel sperm out of the seminiferous tubules. When ultrasound detects ectasia of the rete testis, multiple anechoic cysts will be visualized in the testicular hilum due to obstruction of the efferent ductules. Color flow will not be present in this area of dilation, and this is often seen bilaterally, especially in older men. Sonographers must be able to discern ectasia of the rete testes from any neoplasm that may have internal cystic elements but will also contain solid components.

Hydrocele

A hydrocele is a collection of fluid that forms around the testicle. It is a common problem in newborns and usually resolves itself within the first year of life. It occurs when the testicle descends into the scrotum during fetal development. At this time, the processus vaginalis (from the abdominal cavity) travels along with the testicle. This allows fluid to flow to the scrotum and surround the testicle. By birth, the processus vaginalis typically closes (obliterates) and any remaining fluid is absorbed by the body. If the processus vaginalis remains open, it is called a communicating hydrocele.

Orchitis

Orchitis is the term for an infection that has spread to the testicle. The following ultrasound features are present:

- The testicle may appear normal to enlarged in size.
- Echogenicity of the testicle may be decreased (or heterogeneous).
- Increased blood flow can be observed using color Doppler.
- In cases of chronic orchitis, layers of heterogeneous testicular parenchyma are present.
- Focal orchitis does not affect the epididymis and appears the same as a testicular tumor. The presence of a fever and an increased white blood count are indicative of orchitis.

Testicular Microlithiasis

Testicular microlithiasis is a rare (it occurs in up one-half percent of men) benign condition that causes multiple minute calcifications throughout the testicles. It usually causes no symptoms. In up to eighty percent of cases both testicles are affected. Testicular microlithiasis has been associated with testicular cancer, cryptorchidism (the absence of one or more testicles from the scrotum), infertility and intraepithelial germ cell neoplasia (abnormal tissue growth). The following ultrasound features are present:

- Multiple, echogenic, non-shadowing areas throughout the testicles.
- The calcifications may obscure other features of the testicle.
- An echo-poor (or complex abnormality) within the testicle may indicate the presence of an abscess, orchitis (infection), torsion, or tumor.

Seminoma

Seminomas are cancerous tumors that develop from the germ cells of the testicle (the cells that produce sperm). There are two main types of tumors that are called classical (or typical) seminomas and spermatocytic seminomas. Over ninety five percent of seminomas are classical. They usually affect men in their late thirties to early fifties. The average age of men diagnosed with spermatocytic seminoma is about fifty-five. This is ten to fifteen years older than the average age of men with classical seminomas. Spermatocytic tumors are different from classical seminomas in that they grow very slowly and typically do not spread to other parts of the body. This usually results in a good prognosis for patients diagnosed with spermatocytic seminomas

Primary Testicular Cancer

Up to ninety five percent of primary testicular tumors originate in the germ cells (the cells that produce sperm). Primary testicular cancer typically occurs in men between the ages of fifteen and thirty four. Usually there are no symptoms present, although in some cases (ten to fifty percent) there is acute pain in the scrotal area. Invasive testicular germ cell cancers begin as a noninvasive form of the disease (called carcinoma in situ or intratubular germ cell neoplasia). It takes about five years for carcinoma in situ to progress to the invasive form of germ cell cancer. When testicular cancer becomes invasive, its cells penetrate the surrounding tissues and spread (through blood circulation or lymph nodes) to other parts of the body.

Ultrasound Features of Malignant Testicular Tumors

The following ultrasound features are typically present for malignant testicular tumors:

- The tumors appear as well-defined masses.
- The masses are hypoechoic although they sometimes appear heterogeneous.
- Seminomas take on a hypoechoic appearance and are more homogeneous than nonseminomatous germ cell tumors.
- Choriocarcinoma tumors may have cystic features caused by necrosis and bleeding.
- Tumors of the sex cord stroma (Leydig and Certoli cell tumors) may appear as non-homogeneous testicles.
- Germ cell tumors larger than one half inch typically have many blood vessels and a disorganized blood flow.

Nonseminomatous Germ Cell Tumors

Nonseminomatous germ cell tumors may contain any of the following forms:

- Embryonal cell tumors are characterized by a rapid growth rate and the cancer is spread via the bloodstream and lymph nodes to other parts of the body (such as the lungs and liver). The most common age group affected is twenty to thirty-year olds. Over sixty percent of patients have metastases at the time of presentation. Scrotal pain is a common symptom in these patients.
- Choriocarcinoma is the most aggressive form of nonseminomatous germ cell tumor. It is spread through the bloodstream to the lungs, liver, brain, and other organs very early in the disease process. Bleeding is common in patients with metastatic choriocarcinoma.
- Yolk sac tumors typically present as a large primary tumor and occur most often in infancy and early childhood.

Spermatoceles

Spermatoceles are painless, benign, cysts that usually grow in the head of the epididymis. They can be singular or multiple in number and are usually filled with a milky or clear colored fluid containing nonviable sperm. Over time, spermatoceles may remain constant in size or they may grow. The following ultrasound features are present:

- Spermatoceles appear as cysts, are anechoic with posterior enhancement, and have rounded, well-defined walls.
- Spermatoceles cannot be differentiated from simple cysts of the epididymis (that are filled with clear fluid rather than sperm).
- Simple cysts of the epididymis are much less common than spermatoceles.

Spleen

Anatomic Variants that May Be Visualized When Scanning the Spleen

If the sonographer visualizes a mass located in the splenic hilum, an accessory spleen must be considered. It is a common variant that is a congenital anomaly, and it can be identified as an oval or spherical "mass" that has the same appearance as the tissue found in the spleen. Although the typical location is within the splenic hilum, it may actually be visualized anywhere in the abdominal or pelvic cavity. A wandering spleen occurs when this organ is not in the usual left upper quadrant (LUQ) location. The ligaments that typically hold the spleen in place were not present at birth, which may allow the spleen to migrate from the LUQ. If this occurs, the vessels of the spleen may become twisted and cut off blood supply to it. Another variant includes the shape of the spleen, which can look different from patient to patient and not take on the typical elliptical shape with a concave border inferiorly.

Splenomegaly

Splenomegaly is an enlargement of the spleen. It is highly associated with hypersplenism (an enlarged spleen and a decrease in one or more types of blood cells). Any condition that causes a rapid breakdown of blood cells (such as any of the hemolytic anemias) can place a great strain on the spleen and make it enlarge. Other common causes include portal hypertension, acquired immune deficiency syndrome (AIDS), infiltration of the spleen by leukemia (or lymphoma), and infection. Symptoms of splenomegaly may include an inability to eat a large meal and pain in the upper left side of the abdomen.

Where to Look When Splenomegaly Is Apparent

Other areas to be scanned when the spleen is enlarged would be both the upper and lower quadrants of the abdomen, looking for liver enlargement or liver disease. The ultrasound technician should scan over the areas of the portal veins and the splenic vein. Look for nodes that may be enlarged or masses that may be present causing some kind of obstruction. Look around the area of the gallbladder and pancreas. Look for enlargement or shadows that may suggest or confirm lymphoma. Look at the kidneys and for any signs of hydronephrosis, pancreatitis, obstruction of the ureter, or, in female patients, the ovaries. When scanning one quadrant of the abdomen, it is likely that the sonographer will look around the four quadrants of the abdomen for abnormalities as well as anatomically correct focal points.

Histoplasmosis

Histoplasmosis is a disease caused by the fungus histoplasma capsulatum (a common soil-based fungus found in the central and eastern US). The disease primarily affects the lungs (since the dry fungal spores are usually inhaled). The symptoms are similar to tuberculosis. It can, however affect other organs in the body. This form of the disease is called disseminated histoplasmosis, and it can be fatal (especially if left untreated). Disseminated histoplasmosis is more frequently seen in patients with cancer or AIDS. Using ultrasound, the affected spleen appears with multiple focal, bright, echogenic, granulomatous lesions throughout.

Cysts of the Spleen

Eighty percent of all splenic cysts are pseudocysts (an abnormal structure that resembles a cyst but has no membranous lining). They are usually the result of prior trauma to the spleen. More rarely, they can also be caused by congenital conditions (epidermoid cysts) and parasites (echinococcal). Affected patients typically present with a symptom-free lower upper quadrant mass. The following ultrasound features are present:

- Parasitic cysts appear as anechoic lesions (with possible calcification) or as solid masses (with fine internal echoes and poor distal enhancement).
- True (or primary cysts) are typically solitary and rarely calcified.
- Both types of cysts have well defined walls.

Superficial Structures

Associated Pathology Assessed with Ultrasound

Advancements in high-frequency transducers have enabled ultrasound users to assess superficial structures that could not be properly visualized in the past.

Subcutaneous tissue is fat that is located just under the skin that will have different thicknesses depending on the amount of adipose tissue that the patient has. Lipomas are common masses found in the subcutaneous layer that often appear as elliptical, are compressible, and are typically isoechoic or hyperechoic when compared to the surrounding tissue. When scanning the thyroid, it is important that users are aware of the possibility of a third lobe called the pyramidal lobe. This should not be mistaken for a mass, and it will appear as normal thyroid tissue arising superiorly from the isthmus. Cutaneous hemangiomas are superficial masses that can be evaluated with ultrasound. They will appear as hyperemic masses with borders that are well defined.

Lipomas

Lipomas are common masses that sonographers may be required to scan, although physicians often diagnose these clinically without medical imaging. They are a benign, fatty, elliptical subcutaneous mass that are often compressible and contain echogenic strands running parallel to the skin line. Color Doppler may display a wide array of vascularity. Lipomas may be associated with weight gain, and patients may have more than one lipoma. Lipomas are usually fairly small with a diameter of less than 3 cm, but they can grow into larger masses. Ultrasound is useful to determine the size and location of these masses. Subcutaneous lipomas are the most common type of these masses, and they are often visualized in the proximal portions of the extremities, neck, and back. Lipomas that are deeper may have similar appearances to a sarcoma because these borders are more difficult to visualize and are less compressible. They can be located within, above, below, or between muscles and may need to be evaluated further by magnetic resonance imaging.

Identifying Infections Within Superficial Structures

An abscess is one type of infection that may be diagnosed and evaluated with ultrasound. A physician may choose to drain an abscess under ultrasound guidance once it has been diagnosed. An abscess may have a wide array of appearances, but a collection of fluid that is either anechoic or hypoechoic, often displaying posterior enhancement is suggestive of an abscess. The borders of an abscess may be difficult to discern, and overlying soft tissues may appear edematous. Internal septa, gas, and floating particulates may be seen within the abscess, especially when light pressure is applied. Color or power Doppler will usually show peripheral blood flow or flow within adjacent tissues due to inflammation, but absent internal blood flow. When ultrasound guidance is used for aspiration of an abscess, the fluid should be sent to the lab for confirmation of an infection. A larger needle may be necessary in order to withdraw fluid in the presence of infection.

Necrotizing Fasciitis

Necrotizing fasciitis (NF) is a bacterial infection of the soft tissues that will affect the superficial and deep portions of the fascial planes. NF is rare, but it can be fatal if not treated. Often, patients that contract NF already have a chronic disease such as diabetes. A quick diagnosis can be difficult because in the early stage it may appear similar to cellulitis, but when collections of fluid are located within the deep fascia,

NF is suspected. Cellulitis is a more superficial finding, and if NF is diagnosed early, the skin and muscles may not be affected. NF requires an emergent diagnosis, and ultrasound operators should look for "STAFF," which stands for demonstration of subcutaneous thickening, air, in addition to fascial fluid. Air can be seen when certain bacteria tend to form gas within the tissue that is affected. A high-frequency transducer should be used to better image the fascial plane and gas bubbles that often demonstrate posterior shadowing.

Cellulitis

Cellulitis is an infection often caused by staphylococcus or streptococcus bacteria. Cellulitis may be diagnosed during a physical exam if a patient has edematous changes of the extremities that make the skin look as if it is stretched tightly and feels warm to the touch. It will often be visualized in ultrasounds while scanning extremities to determine if a patient has a deep vein thrombosis, also known as a blood clot. In the early stages, a mix of anechoic fluid and echogenic edematous subcutaneous tissue can be visualized with cellulitis, although ultrasound findings may depend on how severe it is and the length of time that the patient has had it. In cases of worsening cellulitis or in a more advanced state, the ultrasound appearance often resembles a cobblestone road. This is due to the amount of subcutaneous fluid separating the fat within the tissue, and it is a common appearance of swelling in the subcutaneous spaces. Color or power Doppler will often demonstrate hyperemia in tissue in which cellulitis is present.

Ultrasound Imaging to Diagnose Abdominal Mass

First, if a mass is palpated by a physician, the ultrasound is ordered to help determine the depth of the mass and whether it is superficial or deep in the abdominal cavity. The peritoneal fascial line will be universally used as a focal point for diagnosis. The transducer used during the scan can be used to compress the area and displace gas or bowel for a clear image of the mass. The mass can then be clearly marked on the scan with identifying surrounding structures, which allows the physician to look for sonographic characteristics. This can help lead to the identification of cysts, solids, irregular borders, movement of air or fluid, size (by using three-dimensional imaging), and vascularity (by using color and pulsed Doppler).

Ultrasound Findings of Superficial Foreign Bodies

Foreign bodies that are not radiopaque can be difficult to diagnose and are common reasons for malpractice cases because retained objects can lead to complications from infections. The use of high-frequency transducers provides clinicians with better resolution when evaluating superficial structures in situations in which the use of X-ray was not successful in locating the object. Although locating a foreign body depends on the skill of the operator, size, and depth of the object, other clues can be helpful in the location attempt. Inflammation will be evident if the object has been in place for a while. The sonographic appearance of foreign bodies will be hyperechoic and will likely display some sort of artifact (reverberation, comet tail, or shadowing). Edematous tissue or an abscess will be represented by a ring around the object that is hypoechoic. Ultrasound can provide clinicians with important information such as the size of the object, depth, and how close the object is to blood vessels, muscles, tendons, and nerves.

Urinary System

Duplex Collecting System

In a normal urinary tract, each kidney is connected to one ureter that drains urine into the bladder. Patients with a duplex collecting system will have two ureters for one kidney that drain independently into the bladder. This condition often occurs with the distal ureter ballooning at its opening into the bladder, forming a sack-like pouch (called a ureterocele). When a patient has an ureterocele, the portion of the ureter closest to the bladder typically becomes enlarged because the ureter opening is very tiny and obstructs urine outflow. As the urine flow is obstructed, urine backs up in the ureter tube. In a duplex collecting system, the ureter with the ureterocele generally drains the top half of the kidney while the duplicate may drain the lower half. An isolated duplex collecting system may be a completely benign condition and may not require therapy.

Horseshoe Kidney

Horseshoe kidney is an anomaly of the kidney included in a group of called fusion anomalies, in which both kidneys are fused together in early embryonic life. Horseshoe kidney is the most common fusion anomaly. Horseshoe kidney refers to the appearance of the fused kidney, which results from fusion at one pole. In more than ninety percent of cases, fusion occurs along the lower pole. Specifically, the term horseshoe kidney is reserved for cases in which most of each kidney lies on one side of the spine. It includes:

- Symmetric horseshoe kidney (fusion along the midline).
- Asymmetric horseshoe kidney (or L-shaped kidney) when the fused part (the isthmus), lies slightly alongside the midline (lateral fusion).

Junctional Parenchymal Defect

Using ultrasound, a junctional parenchymal defect is observed as a triangle-shaped echogenic area within the upper part (pole) of the kidney. It is best observed using a sagittal plane scan. The defect is formed by extensions of the renal sinus cavity in cases where there is a clear division between the upper and lower poles of the kidney. This division is the result of the way the kidney is formed in the fetus. Two masses of embryonic parenchymatous tissue (renunculi) fuse to form the kidney itself. When there is a partial fusion, the junctional parenchymal defects occur where the original two masses of renunculi joined together. This is an entirely normal and benign condition.

Extrarenal Pelvis

The renal pelvis is the expansion on the upper end of the ureter into which the renal calices open. The renal pelvis is normally situated entirely within the renal sinus. In the case of an extrarenal pelvis, a large part of the renal pelvis lies outside the kidney. The kidney itself will appear longer than normal. In most case this is a benign condition, however, an extrarenal pelvis could indicate that an obstruction of the junction between the ureter and the pelvis is present. The following ultrasound features are present:

- The extrarenal pelvis will appear as a central cystic area that lies outside of the kidney proper.
- A transverse view should be used to observe the connection of the extrarenal pelvis with the renal sinus.

Dromedary Hump

The dromedary hump appears as a distinct bulge-like shape along the side and above the border of the left kidney. In some cases, it may be large and prominent enough to be mistaken for a tumor. It is believed to form due to pressure by the spleen against the upper part of the left kidney during fetal development. The dromedary hump is a benign feature of the left kidney and is completely normal. This is confirmed by the presence of a uniform thickness of the renal parenchyma between the bulge and the underlying normal calyces. The following ultrasound feature is present:

- The ultrasound echogenicity is very similar to the renal cortex.

Solitary Kidney and Pelvic Kidney

A solitary kidney is a rare condition. It occurs when only one kidney is formed (instead of two) during embryonic development due to agenesis (the absence or failed development of a body part). The solitary functioning kidney is typically enlarged, and the remaining "empty" kidney location should be examined for the presence of a small, non-functional kidney. If a kidney is not observed in its normal location, the patient's retroperitoneum and pelvis should be scanned. In most cases the "lost" kidney will be found in the patient's bony pelvis region. Pelvic kidney is a developmental abnormality in which the kidney (or kidneys) is located in pelvis instead of normal abdominal lumbar position in the renal fossa.

Intrinsic Renal Disease

There are two classes of diseases that constitute intrinsic renal disease. The first group produces an increase of cortical echoes due to their deposits of collagen and fibrous tissue. This first list includes:

- Interstitial nephritis: Nephritis in which the connective tissue between the cells is mostly affected.
- Acute tubular necrosis: Acute tubular necrosis is a disease involving the damage and death of the renal tubule cells. It is caused by a lack of oxygen to the kidney (ischemia).
- Amyloidosis: Damage of the kidney caused by deposits of amyloid (a waxy, translucent substance, composed primarily of protein fibers).

- Diabetic nephropathy: Disease of the kidney (caused by diabetes) in which the glomerulus thickens and allows abnormally high levels of protein to be eliminated in the urine.
- Systemic lupus erythematosus: an autoimmune inflammatory disease of the kidney's connective tissues.
- Myeloma: A malignant tumor formed by the cells of bone marrow.

The second group of diseases causes a loss of the ability to distinguish between the renal cortex and medullary regions. This second list includes:

- Chronic pyelonephritis: Long-term inflammation of both the lining of the pelvis and the parenchyma of the kidney.
- Renal tubular ectasia: Dilatation or distension of the renal tubules.
- Acute bacterial nephritis: Episodic inflammation of the kidney caused by a bacterial infection.

Renal atrophy is a common outcome of these diseases. The kidneys take on a highly echogenic enlarged appearance. The renal sinus is enlarged (and appears filled with fat) with a very thin cortical rim. Accumulation of fluid within the kidney (edema) caused by renal vein thrombosis, pyelonephritis, or renal transplant rejection results in an increase in echogenicity and renal enlargement.

Hydronephrosis

Hydronephrosis is any swelling of the kidney due to the back up of urine. The following ultrasound features are usually present:

- A dilated renal pelvis and calices.
- The renal sinus and tissue (parenchyma) become more and more compressed (as the urine backs up) until only tiny cyst-like spaces remain.
- Any congenital obstructions of the ureteropelvic junction (UPJ) can be observed.
- The ureters and bladder should be scanned in order determine if they are dilated. Dilation of these structures may indicate obstruction of the urethra or ureterovesical junction.
- If there is any localized hydronephrosis, it is usually due to stones (calculi), focal masses (tumors), or a duplex collecting system.
- Conducting the scan shortly after urination can help to eliminate false-positive errors due to over-hydration, under-hydration, extrarenal pelvis, and any previous urinary diversion procedures.

Non-Obstructive Hydronephrosis

Fluid-filled areas cause the separation of renal echoes. As pressure builds up within the kidney, the renal parenchyma is compressed. The following conditions can cause hydronephrosis without a physical obstruction:

- The presence of reflux.
- The presence of infection.

- Polyuria (the passing of an excessive quantity of urine).
- Post-obstruction atrophy (a tissue-related blockage following elimination of the physical obstruction).
- During pregnancy the enlarged uterus sometimes compresses the ureter (typically on the right side).
- Some conditions such as extrarenal pelvis, peripelvic cysts, reflux, transient diuresis (an increased output of urine), congenital megacalices, papillary necrosis, renal artery aneurysm, and arterial/venous malformations can lead to false-positive results for hydronephrosis.
- Some conditions such as retroperitoneal fibrosis/necrosis and distal calculi can cause false-negative results.

Acute Renal Failure

Acute renal failure can be caused by the following conditions:

- Acute glomerulonephritis.
- Acute interstitial nephritis.
- Acute tubular necrosis.
- Renal vein thrombosis.
- Renal artery occlusion.
- Urinary outflow obstruction.
- Lack of proper blood flow to the kidneys (hypoperfusion).

The following ultrasound features are present:

- Ultrasound scans can easily differentiate between urinary outflow obstructions (that account for up to five percent of all cases of renal failure) and parenchymal disease.
- When an obstruction occurs, urinary tract dilation is always present. The amount of dilation does not always correlate with the degree of obstruction.
- Post-renal failure is usually associated with cancer of the bladder, prostate, uterus, ovaries, and rectum.
- Less likely causes of post-renal failure are retroperitoneal fibrosis/tumor, paraaortic lymph nodes, renal calculi (kidney stones), and papilla fibers in the urine.

Sinus Lipomatosis

Sinus lipomatosis is the accumulation of a moderate amount of fat in the kidney's sinus region. The kidney's normal sinus is composed of fibrous tissue, fat, lymphatic vessels and vascular structures. The degree of fat infiltration (in the form of fibrofatty tissue) varies by patient. The fibrofatty tissue may cause an enlargement of the sinus region. This condition is usually normal and benign. However, it has been associated with chronic renal infections, abscesses and kidney stones. The following ultrasound features are present:

- The central sinus region may be enlarged and show an increase in echogenicity.
- In the normal kidney, the sinus region appears as a central bright area.

Sickle Cell Nephropathy

Sickle cell nephropathy is a progressive renal disease resulting from red blood cells (in patients suffering from sickle cell anemia) sickling in the renal capillaries. This produces focal areas of bleeding (hemorrhage), necrosis, inflammation, fibrosis, and tubular atrophy. Symptoms may include those commonly tied to renal failure, including hematuria (blood in the urine), urinary tract infections, and polyuria (the passing of an excessive quantity of urine). These abnormalities lead to renal failure and may progress to end-stage renal disease. Similar abnormalities can occur (to a lesser extent) in patients with the sickle cell trait and occasionally lead to kidney failure.

The following ultrasound feature is present:

- If acute renal vein thrombosis is present, the kidneys appear enlarged with deceased echogenicity in the areas secondary to edema.

Review Video: Sickle Cell Disease
Visit mometrix.com/academy and enter code: 603869

Papillary Necrosis

Renal papillary necrosis is a disease of the kidneys involving death of the renal papillae. The renal papillae are the areas of the kidney where the openings from the collecting ducts enter the renal pelvis. Necrosis (tissue death) of this area may make the kidney unable to concentrate the urine. This causes polyuria (the passing of an excessive quantity of urine) and nocturia (frequent urination at night). A complication is that the dead tissue may break off and cause an obstruction of the renal pelvis or ureter. Also, the presence of dead tissue in the urine may cause urinary tract infection. If enough of the renal papillae die, kidney failure will result. Some of the conditions that cause renal papillary necrosis are:

- Sickle cell anemia.
- Renal transplant rejection.
- Urinary tract obstruction.
- Diabetic nephropathy.

AIDS Effect on the Kidneys

Acquired immune deficiency syndrome (AIDS) is a contagious disease passed through intimate contact with various bodily fluids (blood, semen, etc.). It is not passed through casual contact with an infected person. The virus destroys the body's immune defenses by destroying white blood cells (T-Cells). It then replicates widely in the infected person and causes serious damage to many organs. When it attacks the kidneys, uremia (a buildup of toxic urea in the blood) is a common symptom. The following ultrasound features are present:

- There is typically an echogenic pattern in the parenchyma.
- There is an increase in echogenicity of the renal cortex.
- The kidneys appear to be of normal size to somewhat enlarged.

Infections of the Kidneys and Urinary Tract

Infection of the kidneys and urinary tract usually starts as pyelonephritis (the presence of pus in a renal system that has been obstructed for some time). It can then progress to focal bacterial nephritis, and finally turn in an abscess. Ultrasound reveals low-level echoes when there are significant fluid debris levels. Emphysematous pyelonephritis is an infection caused by the presence of air in the kidney parenchyma. It is a very serious condition related to complications from diabetes. Xanthogranulomatous pyelonephritis is a somewhat rare infection related to long-standing urinary tract obstruction. The condition results in damage and destruction of the renal parenchyma. Typical symptoms include renal failure, and the presence of staghorn calculi (kidney stones that involve the renal pelvis and extend into at least 2 calyces). Ultrasound reveals the replacement of normal renal tissue with cystic spaces, diffuse/segmented wave forms, and an enlargement of the affected kidney.

Alport's Syndrome

Alport's syndrome is a chronic nephritis that affects the cell membranes of the kidneys (and often the eyes and ears). This rare, inherited disorder damages the internal structures of the kidney (the glomeruli) and impairs their function by causing glomerulonephritis. Ultimately, this may lead to kidney failure. Alport's syndrome primarily affects males because the genetic defect is on the X chromosome. Typical symptoms include hematuria (blood in the urine), proteinuria (excessive protein in the urine), hypertension, hearing loss, and kidney failure. The following ultrasound features are present:

- Renal cortical echogenicity is increased due to the presence of cellular infiltration and fibrosis in the open gaps and spaces within the kidney.
- The kidneys appear abnormally small.

Lupus Nephritis

Lupus nephritis is an inflammation of the kidney caused by systemic lupus erythematosus. It is a disease of the immune system, and causes inflammation of the skin, joints, kidneys, and brain. The kidneys are affected in more than fifty percent of patients with systemic lupus erythematosus. The disease attacks the glomeruli within the kidney, ultimately causing kidney failure. It occurs in females (more than males) at around thirty years of age. Common symptoms include weight gain, high blood pressure (hypertension), hematuria (blood in the urine), proteinuria (excessive protein in the urine), renal vein thrombosis, and general swelling of the body. The following ultrasound features are present:

- Increased cortical echogenicity.
- Renal atrophy.

Acute Interstitial Nephritis

Acute interstitial nephritis is inflammation the spaces between the tubules (interstitium). It is most often caused by infections (such as those caused by diphtheria and scarlet fever) or side effects of drugs (including allergic reactions). Common symptoms include uremia (accumulation of urea in the blood), proteinuria (excess protein in the urine), hematuria (blood in the urine), eosinophilia (elevation of allergy-fighting white blood cells), rash, and fever. The kidneys become enlarged and mottled, and their function is compromised. The following ultrasound features are present:

- Renal cortical echogenicity is increased.
- If diffuse active disease is present, the increased cortical echogenicity is exaggerated.
- If diffuse scarring is present, the increased cortical echogenicity is subdued.

Acute Glomerulonephritis

In acute glomerulonephritis, the glomerular tissue becomes inflamed. This causes necrosis and excessive cellular growth within the glomeruli. It affects males more than females by a two to one margin. The age of onset is typically five to fifteen years old. Common symptoms include hematuria (blood in the urine), proteinuria (excessive protein in the urine), high blood pressure (hypertension), edema, and impaired renal function. Secondarily, the disease affects the renal vascular elements, tubules, and interstitium. Ultimately, the kidneys become enlarged (up to fifty percent larger than normal) and kidney function is compromised. The following ultrasound features are present:

- There are increased cortical echoes.
- Depending on the source condition causing the glomerulonephritis (membranous, idiopathic, membranoproliferative, rapidly progressive, or poststreptococcal) unique echo patterns emerge.

Transitional Cell Carcinoma

Transitional cell carcinoma is a type of malignant tumor that develops in the lining of the renal pelvis, ureter, or bladder. These tumors are mostly found in the bladder. It is also likely there will be multiple tumors present. Men are more likely to develop these tumors by a three to one ratio. The likelihood of developing transitional cell carcinoma increases with age. The following ultrasound features are present:

- If the tumor is located in the renal pelvis, a mass will be seen with low level echoes, a widening of central sinus echoes, and a hypoechoic central region.
- With this type of tumor, the sonographer may not be able to discern any significant abnormalities.

Renal Cell Carcinoma

Renal cell carcinoma (RCC) is the most common primary renal malignant tumor (neoplasm) in adults. It accounts for eighty five percent of renal tumors and two percent of all adult malignancies. RCC affects men more than women by a two to one margin. It occurs most often in patients fifty to seventy years old. Up to one third of patients already have metastatic disease at the time of presentation. There is a pattern of irregular calcification inside the tumor. Ninety percent of all tumors showing calcification inside the tumor (as opposed to the periphery) are carcinomas. RCCs are staged (using the American Joint Committee on Cancer TNM classification) as follows:

- Stage 1: Confined to the kidney.
- Stage 2: Spread to perinephric fat, but still confined within Gerota's facia.
- Stage 3: Spread to the renal vein, IVC, or lymph node.
- Stage 4: Spread beyond the Gerota fascia, to distant metastases.

Renal Lymphoma

Renal lymphoma is often discovered in patients with known lymphoma. These tumors are often difficult to detect because their infiltrative growth results in preservation of the renal tissue (parenchymal structures) and renal shape. As these tumors enlarge, the surrounding renal parenchyma is compressed and destroyed. Eventually, the renal masses will extend beyond the renal contour and resemble primary renal tumors (neoplasms). Renal involvement occurs more commonly in non–Hodgkin lymphoma than in Hodgkin lymphoma. Patients with renal lymphoma may not have any symptoms, however, the renal function panel occasionally reveals elevated blood urea nitrogen (BUN) and creatinine levels, which may indicate an obstruction. The tumor may obstruct urine flow, resulting in dilation of the branches and pelvic cavity of the kidney due to an accumulation of urine (hydronephrosis).

Mesoblastic Nephroma

Mesoblastic nephroma is the most common benign renal tumor identified in newborn children (the peak age is three months). This tumor is sometimes confused with the congenital Wilms' tumor. It usually occurs in the first six months of life. These tumors can be quite large and take up the entire kidney area. The tumor itself has a homogeneous rubbery appearance, and (unlike Wilms' tumors) is not prone to bleeding. Symptoms may include hematuria, hypertension, vomiting, and hypercalcemia (these are usually seen in a minority of cases). The following ultrasound features are present:

- A large, echogenic mass with a homogeneous echotexture.
- Any heterogeneity may suggest areas of necrosis (tissue death) or bleeding (hemorrhage).

Angiomyolipoma

Angiomyolipoma is a benign renal tumor (neoplasm) composed of fat, vascular, and smooth muscle. It is a rare tumor with an overall incidence of less than one percent.

There are two types of this tumor:

- Isolated angiomyolipoma is usually a small and solitary tumor. It accounts for up to eighty percent of these tumors. The typical patient is a forty-year-old female. The right kidney is involved eighty percent of the time.
- Angiomyolipoma associated with tuberous sclerosis accounts for twenty percent of these tumors. The tumors are larger than isolated angiomyolipoma and there are usually multiple tumors present. Angiomyolipoma occurs in the majority of patients with tuberous sclerosis.

Small angiomyolipoma tumors usually do not cause any symptoms. Larger tumors can result in a palpable mass, hematuria (blood in the urine), and bleeding (hemorrhage) within the tumor.

Renal Adenoma and Oncocytoma

Renal adenoma and oncocytoma are relatively common, benign solid renal tumors. These tumors rarely cause symptoms and are most often incidentally detected through ultrasound and CT scans of the kidney. They appear as small renal masses that are not easily distinguished from renal cell carcinoma. The following ultrasound features are present:

- An adenoma may show differing degrees of calcification.
- An oncocytoma appears as a central scar with surrounding "spokes of a wheel" patterns of enhancement.
- Since these tumors are considered pre-cancerous, the sonographer should look for evidence of spreading to the blood vessels and lymph nodes near the kidney. Any possibilities of malignancy should not be ruled out.

Wilms' Tumor

A Wilms' tumor is the most common renal tumor detected in the pediatric population. These are often found in patients younger than the age of five, with most cases diagnosed when the child is three or four years old. This is the most common malignant cancer diagnosed in childhood. These masses are often noticed by the child's parents because a lump may be felt in the abdomen. The child may also have abdominal pain and/or hematuria (blood in the urine). A Wilms' tumor is also referred to as a nephroblastoma. The ultrasound appearance of a nephroblastoma is a predominantly solid mass found within the kidney that may be heterogeneous in the presence of necrosis or hemorrhage. The tumor may also contain fat or calcifications. It is important to note that a nephroblastoma is typically unilateral, but it may occur in the right and the left kidneys. When a solid mass is present, the sonographer must check the renal vein(s) and inferior vena cava to determine if there is vascular extension of the mass.

Simple Renal Cysts of the Kidneys and Urinary Tract

The exact causes of simple renal cysts are not well known. It is believed to develop after tubular obstruction, vascular occlusion, or focal inflammation. These cysts develop in up to fifty percent of adults over fifty years old. The following ultrasound features are present:

- There are no internal echoes present.
- Acoustic enhancement occurs.
- There is a clear outline of the back wall of the cyst.
- The cyst is spherical or slightly ovoid in shape.
- Low-level echoes originating from the cyst may be due to an artifact (sensitivity is set too high or a transducer frequency that is too low), infection, hemorrhage, a necrotic cystic tumor, or technique (a high amount of reverberation from the back wall of the cyst).

Von-Hippel-Lindau Cysts of the Kidneys and Urinary Tract

Von Hippel-Lindau syndrome is an inherited condition that manifests itself by forming fluid-filled cysts throughout the body. The cysts usually form during young adulthood, however, the signs and symptoms related to the presence of the cysts may occur at any age. Patients afflicted with this syndrome commonly develop cysts in the kidneys and pancreas.

Renal adenomas can also form and may turn cancerous (renal adenocarcinoma).

A unique tumor called a hemangioblastoma is characteristic of von Hippel-Lindau syndrome. The tumor is usually located in the brain (or eyes) and is composed of newly formed blood vessels. It is mostly non-cancerous; however, it may cause complications depending on where the tumor is located within these organs.

Atypical Cysts and Para-Pelvic Cysts of the Kidneys and Urinary Tract

Atypical cysts are cysts that tend to show bleeding (hemorrhage). Ultrasound shows low-level echoes, multiple divisions (septae), and echoes within the cyst. Some (up to three percent) show mural nodules or rim-shaped calcification. Of these, up to twenty percent may be malignant.

Para-pelvic cysts show up in the renal hilum, but do not spread to the urine collecting system. Symptoms may include flank pain, high blood pressure (hypertension), and symptoms related to obstructions (such as acute renal failure). Ultrasound shows no divisions (septations). There may be irregular borders due to distortion of the renal sinus structures (caused by compression). The cyst may cause an obstruction of the renal system.

Multi-Cystic Dysplastic Kidney

Multi-cystic dysplastic kidney is the most common palpable mass found in neonates. It is a congenital condition that is not hereditary. Usually, only one kidney is involved. In infants, the kidney appears enlarged and is non-functioning. In adults, the affected kidney may appear smaller than normal with significant calcification. Large, multiple cysts are usually seen that cover the entire parenchyma. This results in a "cluster of grapes" appearance of the kidney. To rule out hydronephrosis, the sonographer must be able to show connection to the renal pelvis. Some associated complications are:

- Urethral atresia (congenital unconnected, or absent, ureter).
- A non-functioning kidney.
- Atretic renal artery (congenital unconnected, or absent, renal artery).

Tuberous Sclerosis and Acquired Cystic Disease of Dialysis

Tuberous sclerosis (Bourneville's disease) is a congenital disease that causes multiple renal cysts. Typically, there are also multiple renal angiomyolipomas (benign tumors composed of fatty (adipose) tissue, muscle cells, and vascular structures). The typical patient afflicted with this disease has a history of seizures, mental deficiency, and skin tumors.

Patients that require long-term dialysis have a greater chance of developing renal cysts. Up to ninety percent of dialysis patients show some signs of renal cystic disease after two to three years of treatment. These cysts sometimes bleed (hemorrhage). These patients also have an increased incidence of renal adenomas and cancer (up to seven times greater than the general population).

Multilocular Cystic Nephroma

Multilocular cystic Nephroma is a rare benign cystic renal tumor. It is not hereditary, and the cause is not well understood. It most often occurs in boys up to four years old, and women who are over thirty years old. It typically affects only one kidney and appears as a solitary multiloculated cyst. The cyst is lined with epithelial cells and there are multiple cystic spaces within the tumor (that are separated by fibrous septa). The tumor does not communicate with the renal pelvis, however, it can bulge (herniated) into the renal pelvis. Hydronephrosis may occur due to compression of the renal collecting system. Up to ten percent of these cysts show calcification.

Medullary Cystic Kidney

Medullary cystic kidney is a rare disease that causes chronic interstitial nephritis and fibrosis of the renal medulla. It is not hereditary and typically not seen in children. The renal collecting ducts and tubules can become obstructed due to fibrosis. Calcification occurs in up to eighty percent of affected patients. The cysts themselves are very small (about one twelfth of an inch). Urinary sediments are common (which is rare in cystic disease of the kidney). The condition may cause salt-wasting nephropathy in young adults.

The following ultrasound features are present:

- The kidneys appear smaller than normal.
- There is an increase in echogenicity (causes the renal pyramids to blend with sinus fat).

Color Doppler for Evaluation of the Urinary Bladder

If a mass is visualized in the urinary bladder, it should be documented with gray-scale ultrasound, measurements should be performed, it should be characterized as a mobile or a nonmobile filling defect, and it should be examined with color Doppler. If a solid mass is present, it is helpful in reaching a diagnosis to determine the vascularity of the mass. Blood clots or fungal balls when visualized in the bladder will not demonstrate color flow. Color Doppler may also be useful when evaluating the ureteral jets. The ureteral jets show the urine entering the bladder from the ureters. They are not always visible with gray-scale, so they can be examined more closely with color Doppler for diagnostic confidence as the bladder is filling. If after several minutes one of the jets is not visualized, it may indicate an obstruction of the ureter on that side. If stones are identified within the bladder, it may be useful to determine if "twinkling artifacts" are present when color Doppler is used.

Vascular Abnormalities

Cavernous Hemangioma

Cavernous hemangioma is small tumor (about one inch). It is the most common benign liver tumor with an occurrence of 0.4 to 7.3 percent in the general population. Cavernous hemangioma typically occurs on the right lobe of the liver and originates with the endothelial cells that line the blood vessels. Walls made of collagen support its structure and the lesion itself consists of multiple, large vascular channels lined by a single layer of endothelial cells. In most cases, these tumors are without symptoms and discovered upon imaging, surgery, or autopsy. They can occur at any age and are more common in women (by about a five to one margin). When symptoms do occur, they are most likely caused by the compression of adjacent structures, rupture, or acute thrombosis.

Portal Hypertension

Portal hypertension is the buildup of pressure in the portal vein (the vein connecting the intestines and the liver). Normally, the pressure is low compared with the arterial pressure, but slightly above the pressure in the other veins of the body. The most common cause of portal hypertension is liver disease (such as cirrhosis). Portal hypertension usually causes moderate splenomegaly and dilated, tortuous blood vessels at the splenic hilum. It also causes dilation of the portal vein itself. If portal hypertension is suspected, the liver and portal vein should be examined along with the spleen.

Congenital Anomalies of Vessels that May Be Discovered During Abdominal Ultrasound

Congenital anomalies of the blood vessels located in the retroperitoneum are typically an incidental finding during an ultrasound exam. It is important to document any variants of the inferior vena cava, aorta, and their branches because critical injuries may occur during abdominal or pelvic surgeries. Although most patients may not have any associated issues with these variants, a diagnosis of congenital anomalies may explain symptoms for those patients that experience hematuria, display a left-sided varicocele, or have pain in the left flank region. These symptoms could be explained if the left renal vein is located posterior to the aorta. A retroaortic left renal vein may prevent adequate drainage of the blood from the left kidney because this vessel is being compressed between the aorta and spine. Another variant is the duplication of renal arteries and veins.

Abdominal Aortic Aneurysm

Ultrasound is often the first modality chosen in the detection of abnormalities of the retroperitoneum due to the low cost and the fact that it does not use ionizing radiation. Ultrasound exams can provide a quick method for detecting an abdominal aortic aneurysm (AAA). The abdominal aorta can be examined by gray-scale, color, and spectral Doppler in patients that are experiencing abdominal or flank pain, when a pulsatile mass is detected in the abdomen, or if a clinician hears an abdominal bruit. Ultrasound is typically the method of choice to follow up an AAA when detected by previous imaging exams or modalities. Any measurement that is greater than or equal to 3 cm in diameter in the infrarenal portion of the aorta is considered to be aneurysmal. This region is also considered to be positive for an aneurysm when the diameter is 1.5 times greater than the segment that is proximal to the renal arteries; this is a great guideline to follow especially in patients that are smaller than average.

Aortic Dissection

An aortic dissection is a life-threatening condition in which the innermost layer of the aorta tears and allows blood to pool between the inner and middle layers of the arterial wall. Although dissections are a fairly uncommon occurrence, they can be difficult to diagnose without medical imaging because the symptoms can mimic a heart attack. Patients may complain of sudden, excruciating chest or abdominal pain that radiates to the back or down the leg and shortness of breath. The quicker that the diagnosis can be made, the better the chances of survival for the patient. Bedside sonography can provide a quick, noninvasive look at the aorta. If an intimal flap is seen within the lumen of the abdominal aorta, a dissection is assumed, and the patient must be sent to surgery immediately. If the outer layer of the aorta ruptures because of the pooling of blood, the patient will typically die.

Using Ultrasound to Determine a Thrombus in the Inferior Vena Cava

Ultrasound is a cost-effective and noninvasive tool that can be used to quickly diagnose medical emergencies. Ultrasound can be performed bedside so that the patient does not have to be taken to the radiology department. The inferior vena cava (IVC) is located to the right of the abdominal aorta, and it returns blood from the lower body to the right atrium of the heart. The IVC is formed when the right and left common iliac veins join within the retroperitoneum. A thrombus (blood clot) may be readily identified in the IVC because it appears as an echogenic filling defect within the lumen of the IVC; a blood clot within the IVC is life-threatening. Color Doppler can also be used to demonstrate the incomplete saturation of color within the vessel. A thrombus in the IVC is typically the result of a deep vein thrombosis of the legs. An IVC filter may be placed in patients that cannot take anticoagulants to prevent emboli from lodging within the lungs or heart.

Thyroid Abnormalities that May Be Diagnosed with Color Doppler Ultrasound

The thyroid gland is vascular; it is supplied by four thyroid arteries (two supply the superior lobes, and two supply the inferior portion of the lobes). During a thyroid ultrasound, the sonographer may notice hyperemia (increased vascularity than normal) of the thyroid gland once color or power Doppler is applied. This is often seen in patients with Graves' disease, which, in the United States, is the most common form of hyperthyroidism (too many thyroid hormones are produced) and is considered to be an autoimmune disorder. When scanning the region of the neck lateral to the thyroid gland, the sonographer may incidentally observe a stenosis in the carotid artery or a blood clot (thrombus) in the jugular vein. Color Doppler is helpful to determine the extent of both of these findings.

Sonographic Appearances of Testicular Torsion

Sonographers should be aware that a gray-scale ultrasound of a testicular torsion may be unremarkable in the first couple of hours after the torsion has occurred. This is the reason why it is important to also evaluate the testes with color, power, and spectral Doppler. If there is a partial torsion or if torsion is taking place during an exam, the ultrasound operator may still see blood flow, but the waveform may not show diastolic flow (or it will be reversed or will be less than normal). Color Doppler may show flow in the testis that is twisted, but it will have the color flashing, which demonstrates absent diastolic flow. In this case, it would be helpful to have the radiologist present or to take a cine clip of a side-by-side comparison with color flow Doppler turned on. The epididymis should also be evaluated with gray-scale and color Doppler because it will not demonstrate blood flow, but it may be enlarged. The scrotal wall may be thickened when torsion has taken place, and the testis may appear hypoechoic. The testes should be measured to determine enlargement. The head, body, and tail of the epididymis should also be examined with gray-scale and color Doppler.

Varicocele

A varicocele is a mass of enlarged veins that develops in the spermatic cord. The spermatic cord is made up of blood vessels, lymphatic vessels, nerves, and the duct that carries sperm from the body (vas deferens). If the valves that regulate blood flow from these veins become defective, blood does not circulate out of the testicles efficiently, which causes swelling in the veins above and behind the testicles. It usually occurs only in the left testicle since the left spermatic vein drains into the renal vein between the superior mesenteric artery and the aorta. These two arteries can compress the renal vein and thus impede blood flow from the spermatic vein. The condition is also associated with infertility. The following ultrasound feature is present:

- Varicoceles appear as a collection of tortuous tubular structures.

Infarction of the Spleen

Infarction of the spleen is usually caused by infection or a blood clot. Several conditions that may cause infarction of the spleen include pancreatitis, endocarditis, leukemia/lymphoma, and sickle cell anemia. Its ultrasound appearance is dependent on when the infarct occurs. A fresh infarct (hemorrhagic) appears hypoechoic. A healed infarct (with scarring) appears as an echogenic, wedge-shaped lesion. The affected patient will usually present with pain in the upper left quadrant of the abdomen. Additional symptoms may include fever, chills, nausea, vomiting, chest pain (upon breathing), and left shoulder pain. Splenic abscess may result, especially if the infarct was caused by an infection.

Benign Tumors of the Spleen

There are three main types of benign tumors that affect the spleen. They are:

- Hamartomas: A common benign tumor of the spleen composed of splenic tissue that grows in a disorganized mass. They are usually asymptomatic. On ultrasound, they appear as well-defined hyperechoic solid masses.
- Cavernous hemangiomas: These tumors are made up jumbled growths of blood vessels fed by numerous tributary arteries. They typically go through a growth phase followed by a rest phase (during which they virtually disappear). They only cause symptoms if they bleed or increase the size of the spleen enough to affect other organs. On ultrasound, they usually appear as a large echogenic mass with small hypoechoic areas.
- Cystic lymphangiomas: A rare benign congenital tumor. It appears as a mass with extensive cystic replacement of the normal splenic tissue.

Malignant Tumors of the Spleen

There are three main types of cancerous tumors that affect the spleen. They are:

- Hemangiosarcoma: This is an aggressive form of cancer. It is a blood-fed sarcoma (the blood vessels grow directly into the tumor and it is typically filled with blood). A frequent cause of death is the rupture of the tumor (which causes severe bleeding). On ultrasound, the tumor has a mixed cystic pattern.
- Lymphoma: Any of the various malignant tumors (of lymphatic and reticuloendothelial tissues) that occur as circumscribed solid tumors. They are composed of cells that resemble lymphocytes, plasma cells, or histiocytes.

- Metastases: Cancer that has spread from other organs of the body. The spleen is the tenth most common site for this type of cancer. It appears (on ultrasound) as multiple, hyperechoic lesions.

Importance of Identifying the Location of the Left Renal Vein

Ultrasound is a cost-effective modality to examine patients that present with symptoms such as fevers, hematuria, urinary tract infections, flank or inguinal pain, or varicoceles. Ultrasound is often the first step in diagnosing any abnormalities of the urinary system. Multiple congenital variations of the left renal vein may occur in which it is positioned behind the aorta and in front of the spine. Although a rare phenomenon, this is known as a retroaortic left renal vein, and symptoms arise because compression increases the pressure of the renal vein. Symptoms such as hematuria are often exasperated by physical activity. Color Doppler is helpful in tracking the renal vein from the kidney to the inferior vena cava, and sonographers may notice that the left renal vein tends to have a smaller diameter when it courses anteriorly to the spine. It is important to note this finding in symptomatic patients or those that are having any type of renal surgery.

Evaluating Urinary System for Vascular Abnormalities Using Doppler Ultrasound Methods

Renal artery stenosis occurs when there is stenosis (narrowing) of the renal arteries. This is typically caused by atherosclerosis, and if left untreated it may cause hypertension or renal failure. A renal artery duplex exam may be ordered to determine the cause of uncontrolled or sudden-onset hypertension, determine the cause of an abdominal bruit, follow up from abnormal lab values or prior imaging studies, or if an aneurysm is suspected. A renal artery duplex includes gray-scale, color, and spectral Doppler interrogation of the abdominal aorta, kidneys, renal arteries, and veins, as well as the smaller vessels within the kidneys. These arteries include the segmental, interlobar, arcuate, and interlobular arteries. The direction of blood flow and turbulence should be documented along with the measurement of peak and end diastolic velocities, resistive index, and pulsatile index.

Trauma

Abnormalities Related to Traumatic Events

Ultrasound can be a great tool to quickly evaluate the presence of free fluid in post-traumatic injuries. Clinicians can use the Focused Assessment with Sonography for Trauma method to help determine the best care for the patient without having to expose them to radiation. This is especially important in children, women that are pregnant, or when multiple victims are sent to the emergency department at once. Physicians and sonographers can evaluate the chest, abdominal, and pelvic cavities for evidence of a pericardial or pleural effusion, pneumothorax, or ascites. Ultrasound may also aid in the diagnosis of an injury involving the liver, spleen, and/or kidneys. The inferior vena cava may also be imaged when the patient has lost a lot of blood. Sonographers should be aware that anechoic fluid visualized within the abdomen or pelvis when the patient is status post-trauma is likely due to a hemorrhage. However, blood may vary in appearance and may even be difficult to discern from the normal surrounding tissue of the solid organs.

Liver Hematomas

Liver hematomas typically occur when there is trauma to the liver. A hematoma occurs when there is bleeding outside of a blood vessel, but the bleeding is contained within the surrounding tissue. It commonly appears as a pooling of blood (usually clotted), which is confined between the capsule (surrounding the liver and known as Glisson's capsule) and the surface of the liver. However, it is possible for a hematoma to occur anywhere there are blood vessels within the liver. Hematomas usually resolve themselves with time and do not require any intervention. In very rare circumstances, a liver hematoma can become very large and rupture into the peritoneal cavity creating a very serious condition for the patient.

Post-Traumatic Sonographic Findings of the Scrotum

B-mode and color Doppler ultrasound is the first imaging modality used for patients that present with scrotal injuries. Clinicians can quickly determine if surgery is necessary in order to preserve the testis. Testicular rupture can be diagnosed if the operator visualizes an interruption of the tunica albuginea. The normal ultrasound appearance should display two echogenic lines that are parallel to each other. When ruptures are present, often the underlying testicular tissue will demonstrate an irregular shape and heterogeneous appearance. Color Doppler should also be used to determine blood flow characteristics because a rupture typically results in interruption of blood flow to at least part of the testicle. A bilateral comparison of blood flow should be documented so that physicians can quickly determine if a rupture or torsion has occurred. A fracture of the testicle will appear as a straight, hypoechoic line that does not display blood flow. The epididymis may also be affected during trauma and will often appear enlarged and hyperemic.

Trauma to the Spleen

Blunt abdominal trauma is the most common reason for injury to the spleen. Motor vehicle accidents are the primary cause (accounting for up to thirty percent of cases). Additionally, any of the diseases (such as portal hypertension) that cause splenic enlargement may cause the spleen to rupture. The affected patient usually presents with upper left quadrant pain. Hypotension and a decreased hemoglobin level may indicate internal bleeding.

The following ultrasound features are present:

- Splenomegaly with progressive enlargement and an irregular splenic border.
- Focal hematomas are represented by intrasplenic fluid collections.
- Sub-capsular hematomas show perispleic fluid collections.
- Blood exhibits various echo patterns (depending on the age of the injury).

- Focal areas show tiny lacerations that give rise to small collections of blood interspersed with disrupted pulp (contusion).
- When the spleen heals (and returns to normal) small, irregular foci may remain.

Rectus Sheath Hematoma

The rectus sheath is made up of the rectus abdominis muscle (a paired muscle running vertically on each side of the front wall of the abdomen), a surrounding facial sheath, and the blood supply from the epigastric arteries and veins. When the rectus abdominis muscle contracts, the attached artery must move with the muscle to avoid tearing. During strong contractions of the rectus abdominis muscles (such as those during rigorous exercise), the artery may tear resulting in a hematoma. External trauma to the abdominal wall may also cause the condition. Abdominal pain in the region of the affected rectus abdominis muscle is usually present.

Abnormalities that May Be Visualized in the Urinary System after a Traumatic Event

In patients that are seen in the emergency department (ED) for trauma-related injuries, ultrasound is a relatively quick and easy method to determine the presence of free fluid within the abdomen and pelvis. An ultrasound can be performed in the ED so that an unstable patient does not have to be moved. Blunt trauma is more often the cause of injury when compared to penetrating forces involving the urinary system. Sonographers should be aware that if injuries are diagnosed in the kidneys due to trauma, the majority of cases will also include other organs. Computed tomography (CT) is often ordered when the patient presents with symptoms causes by trauma to the urinary system because ultrasound cannot diagnose all injuries, especially parenchymal involvement. Ureters are not often visualized due to bowel gas, but ultrasound operators should evaluate the urinary bladder. Rupture of the urinary bladder is better diagnosed with CT, but ultrasound may provide useful information pertaining to free fluid within the abdominopelvic cavity. Ureteral jets may be visualized with color Doppler if a distended urinary bladder is present to rule out the presence of an obstructed ureter.

Postoperative

Ultrasound Examination of Renal Transplant Patient

The following conditions should be looked for:

- Any swelling of the kidney due to the back up of urine (hydronephrosis).
- Fluid collections (such as lymphocele). Lymphoceles are the most common fluid collections in the transplant population (occurring in five to fifteen percent of patients). They are most frequently associated with obstruction of the urethra. On ultrasound, these collections may appear heavily septated and large.

- Any bleeding (hemorrhage). Perinephric hematomas account for twenty-five to thirty percent of all complications. While most are small and do not require additional therapy, haematomas may occasionally compress the ureter and produce hydronephrosis.
- Any signs of acute (or diffuse) infection and acute tubular necrosis (ATN).
- Any signs of rejection (increased size, prominent hypoechoic medullary pyramids, obliteration of the renal sinus fat, or thickening of the renal pelvis).

Technique to Scan Transplanted Kidney

Select a transducer with the highest frequency for depth penetration, usually a 5-MHz one is adequate. A curved transducer gives a large field allowing for accurate length measurements of the entire kidney. Using the postoperative scar helps to locate the transplanted kidney. Long axis views of the kidney will appear along the axis of the scar and the transverse view of the kidney will be at a right angle to the scar. The urinary bladder will be scanned. If the bladder is full of urine, voiding may make what appears as hydronephrosis disappear when scanned again. Color Doppler may be helpful to image flow of blood to and from the transplanted kidney.

Pre- and Post-Surgical Ultrasound Examination for Liver Transplant

Ultrasound is a very useful tool in the pre and post-operative evaluation of the liver patient. Prior to surgery ultrasound is used to evaluate:

- The health of liver tissue (hepatocytes).
- Identify lesions.
- Determine the openness and size of the portal vein, hepatic veins, and the inferior vena cava (IVC).
- Assess the biliary system for dilation.

After surgery, blood clot formation in the hepatic artery (thrombosis) is the most dangerous complication. Ultrasound is used to monitor the health of the hepatic vascular structures after surgery. Thrombosis of the hepatic artery or portal vein may lead to massive death of liver cells (hepatic necrosis). The presence of air in the hepatic parenchyma (functional cells of the liver) shows up as shadowing on the sonogram. Gangrene of the liver is also apparent in the hepatic texture. Some other things to monitor for are portal vein thrombosis and any blockages of the IVC and hepatic veins.

Thyroidectomy

Sonographers will often be asked to image the neck after a thyroidectomy. If prior scans are available, be sure to acquire them and the reports for comparison. A complete history is important to determine why the thyroid was removed and which lobes. It is important to document multiple images of the thyroid bed in the longitudinal and transverse planes. The sonographer should also scan the lateral neck region, and any enlarged lymph nodes, cysts, or masses should be captured with B-mode (with measurements) and color or power Doppler. If a patient is status postsurgical for cancer of the head or neck, it is important to scan all of the various neck regions. Again, if abnormal lymph nodes are visualized, they should be documented and measured. It is important for sonographers to look at the shape of the node (round is abnormal); loss of fatty hilum and cystic or calcified areas are also considered abnormal. The exam should consist of documentation of the vascularity of the node with color or power Doppler.

Transjugular Intrahepatic Portosystemic Shunt

A transjugular intrahepatic portosystemic shunt is placed between the hepatic and portal veins to alleviate the pressure in the portal system that may be causing ascites or variceal bleeding. In patients that have severe portal hypertension, the flow of blood within the portal venous system tends to be in a hepatofugal direction (flowing away from the liver) instead of hepatopetal (flowing toward the liver). After the stent is placed, a baseline ultrasound should be performed to check the shunt with B-mode and color Doppler. When color Doppler is applied, the entire stent should demonstrate complete color filling. If the ultrasound operator does not see color flow, then one can assume that there is a blockage. If spectral waveforms demonstrate velocities that are extremely high or low when compared to the baseline exam, one may assume that there is a stenosis. Other indicators that the stent is no longer working correctly are a shift in directional flow within the portal vein, ascites that has increased, or the presence of collateral channels visualized with ultrasound.

Physics

Necessary Skills Needed to Master Proper Sonographic Techniques

It is understood that the sonographer has basic knowledge of anatomy, sonographic data, and disease processes. The technician must also do more than just know the basics of the equipment, the transducers, and the way to record the images. The sonographer today must have a vast knowledge of the disease process, the understanding of conditions that require a special technique or unique view to be conclusive, and how to prepare the patient in the case of any special last-minute scanning procedures to ensure a proper diagnosis. They must be able to compile clinical data, review charts, obtain a patient history, and to put all of that together to help form the clinical picture. Then the sonographer must use critical thinking to help get the best images from each individual patient to make the right diagnosis. Each patient differs in body make, weight, age, and the technician must put it all together to make the best use of the scan to get the best images.

Physics Principles in Sonography

There are three categories to evaluate sound. Infrasound is below 20 Hz and humans cannot hear it. Audible sound is between 20 Hz and 20,000 Hz. Ultrasound beams are above 20,000 Hz and are above human hearing ability. Sound waves travel at a variety of speeds and depths depending on pressure, density, and particle motion of the sound energy. Matter has to be present for sound to travel as it cannot go through a vacuum. The waves of sound carry energy from one place to another and vibrations from one molecule carry to the next molecule in the same axis. These movements of sound will continue until friction or something causes it to stop. Sound waves contain areas of high pressure called compression and low pressure called rare-fraction on each wave. Wavelength variability is determined by propagation of speed, period of time in which the cycle occurs, and frequency or number of cycles in one second. All but the propagation of speed can be determined by the transducer. Stiffness and density of the tissue or medium is what determines the propagation of speed.

Choosing a Scanning Technique

No matter which transducer is used or which examination is being performed, certain principles apply. The sound beam should be as perpendicular to the structure being scanned as possible unless it is a Doppler examination. Always scan through the best sound window possible, like liver, bladder, or mass. Often it may be necessary to have the patient fill the bladder by drinking to offer that optimum window. Always demonstrate the long axis whenever possible and then turn 90 degrees to show the short axis. Don't be careless when photographing an image that may be an artifact when suspecting pathology may be present. Make the image as clear as possible before taking the image. Select the best transducer for the job to get the best image using the highest frequency that will penetrate the tissue without putting the gain at the highest limit. Currently, color is used to demonstrate fluid motion or flow.

Transducer

There are several different types of transducers for different types of exams both external and internal. The basic physics design on the inside is the same, but the contour and size may differ for the type of examination being done. There are small parts transducers to do very small areas or for infants and neonates. These types of small transducers will offer a better image than a normal sized transducer would when attempting to scan a very small area like between the ribs. Rectal transducers are made in longitudinal or linear and transverse or radial configurations. These are made specifically to enter the rectum and to image from that angle. Biopsy transducers allow for imaging as well as allowing the availability to obtain biopsy under visual guidance. Doppler probes allow for imaging within a vessel or duct. Transesophageal transducers allow for imaging from the esophagus and seeing the heart.

The transducer has five parts, a crystal, the matching layers, damping material, the transducer case, and the electric cable. The crystal converts the electrical voltage into sound energy to transmit and then reverses the sound energy into electrical energy when the sound beam returns or echoes back to the transducer. The matching layers lie before the transducer element and make the acoustic connection between the skin and the transducer. The damping material, such as rubber, acts as insulation and decreases extra vibrations. The transducer case houses the entire crystal, damping material, and insulation from interference with the electrical noise. The electrical cable contains the wires to conduct and transmit the electrical impulses from circuit source.

The linear array transducer provides the image in a rectangle. It is used when ultrasounding small parts and for vascular imaging. Some linear array transducers can be used for beam steering, giving the ability to guide the gray scale picture more accurately. A trapezoid image shape can be displayed as well from a linear array, making the visual format wider and better for attaining measurements. A vector transducer also gives a trapezoid image and is useful in gynecological, obstetrical, and abdominal examinations. The sector picture is pie shaped, lending itself to cardiac, transcranial, and obstetrical examinations. The curved array allows for a large field of vision and is more commonly used in obstetrics.

Linear array is a format offering a rectangular image of an area. It is most useful in small parts of the anatomy and in vascular imaging. It may offer additional formatting in beam steering and in virtual format, offering the ability to look at a trapezoid image shape which will give a wider view of the area. The Vector format offers a trapezoid image shape as well and is often used in abdominal, gynecological, and obstetric exams. The sector image is pie shaped and can be used in cardiac or abdominal imaging. The curved array provides a large field of view helpful in abdominal or obstetrical imaging. Advances in equipment and the development of specific transducers and formats help imaging to be specific and accurate.

Linear Array Transducer and Phased Array Transducer

In a linear array transducer, multiple crystals are positioned along the face of the transducer in a linear fashion. This forms an ultrasound beam that appears as a rectangle on the sonogram monitor. It also provides for a larger near field of view.

In a phased array transducer, the sequence in which the crystals are fired is electronically controlled in a way that allows the ultrasound beam to be steered and focused. Phased array transducers can be used to generate both sector and rectangular shaped images on the sonogram monitor.

Best Transducer for Small-Parts Scanning

Linear sequential (switched) transducers are the best choice for small-parts ultrasound exams. The design of the probe, which is long and narrow, allows for easier skin contact of the area being interrogated because these regions of the body are often smaller or more difficult to reach. The shape that results from this probe is rectangular, which is the most appropriate because sector images provide a wide field of view in the far field that is not necessary with these types of exams. The lateral resolution changes with scanning depth, but it is better in the far field because these probes have higher frequencies. Of course, the lateral resolution is the best at the focal point where the beam is the absolute narrowest, so the best way to optimize the lateral resolution is to use the highest number of focal zones.

Most Basic Form of Real-Time or Gray-Scale Imaging

The most basic form of real-time or gray-scale imaging is known as brightness mode. This method is more commonly referred to as B-mode imaging. B-mode was the first gray-scale imaging method available. During B-mode, pulses are sent into the body and when the signal returns it appears as a dot on the screen. The amplitude or strength of the reflectors will be visualized as dots. Higher amplitudes will appear as bright-white areas on the screen. The areas that return weaker signals will be discerned as a gray dot on the image display. Even when color mode is used, the underlying image showing the actual anatomy of the patient is represented by gray-scale imaging.

Parameters Increased When Increasing the Output Power

Increasing the output power will have an impact on many parameters. One impact is that the sonographer will be afforded the opportunity to penetrate deeper in the body of the patient. Another parameter that is adjusted is the brightness of the image. When the output power is increased, the image becomes brighter throughout the entire display. If the output power is decreased, the overall image becomes darker. Increasing the output power will force the pulser component of the ultrasound machine to increase the amount of voltage that the PZT crystals receive in the transducers. This will create stronger pulses that are sent into the tissue, which in turn, creates an image that is brighter because of the amplified signals. It is important to note that output power is also referred to as acoustic power or output gain.

Fundamental Frequency and Harmonic Frequency

The fundamental frequency is the actual frequency that is being imparted from the ultrasound transducer and passed into the patient. This is also known as the transmitted frequency. Sometimes the ultrasound beam is altered and creates exams that are not of diagnostic quality. Modern ultrasound systems offer harmonic imaging to help increase diagnostic confidence in those difficult studies. If a sonographer uses harmonic ultrasound, the harmonic frequency used is two times higher than the fundamental (transmitted) frequency. The sound beam is altered less, and the harmonic ultrasound beam helps improve diagnostic capabilities. Tissue and contrast harmonics are two examples of the types of harmonic ultrasound used today.

Applications of Harmonic Imaging During Abdominal Ultrasounds

Tissue harmonics are not contained within the ultrasound beam that is emitted from the transducer. Tissue harmonics are produced when the sound beam interacts with tissues that are deeper in the body in a nonlinear fashion. With this being said, tissue harmonics do not occur when the scanning depth is shallow. These sound beams that are being transmitted must be strong; weak sound waves will not produce any tissue harmonics at all. With strong beams, the harmonics are created within the main line of the ultrasound wave. Tissue harmonics will only emerge from this main axis and will create very few imaging errors because of the strength of the beam. Harmonic frequencies allow the sonographer to scan patients at higher frequencies that will improve not only the axial resolution, but the lateral resolution as well. The lateral resolution tends to improve because the wave is more narrow (higher frequency beams produce a narrower beam). Harmonics are enabling sonographers to see organs that are deeper in the body, as well as eliminating reverberation artifacts in organs such as the gallbladder. The reverberation artifacts can mimic sludge within the gallbladder.

Advantages and Disadvantages of Power Doppler

Power Doppler (also referred to as energy mode or color angio) is a form of color Doppler that does not display the speed of blood flow or any directional information. Rather, it only determines that a Doppler shift has taken place and shows the amplitude of the moving blood. If there are more red blood cells in one area, the signals will be brighter. Vessels represented with power Doppler will all be identical colors on the display. Advantages of power Doppler include the fact that aliasing does not occur because the speed and direction of blood flow is not applicable. Power Doppler picks up blood flow in smaller vessels and slow blood flow because of its increase in sensitivity. There is an increase in sensitivity because power Doppler is not altered by the Doppler angle. A disadvantage of power Doppler is that, due to the increased sensitivity, flash artifact may be visualized when the patient moves or breathes. Power Doppler does not evaluate the direction or velocity of blood flow. When compared to color Doppler, the temporal resolution is greatly reduced.

Sampling Velocities at a Chosen Location During a Pulsed-Wave Doppler Exam

When performing a pulsed-wave Doppler exam, the user is able to determine exactly where a velocity measurement should be taken within a vessel. Once the sonographer has the grayscale image optimized, color Doppler can be activated to better visualize the blood vessels. Then, one can bring up the cursor for pulsed-wave Doppler and a line that is intersected by two dashes close together will be visualized. This is the gate (sample volume). The gate can be moved with the trackball until it is right where the user wants to perform a spectral analysis. The size of the gate can be changed so that it is only within the vessel that is being examined. For example, if one is sampling the carotid artery but the spectral display is also showing venous flow, reduce the size of the gate and reposition it so that only the artery is being interrogated.

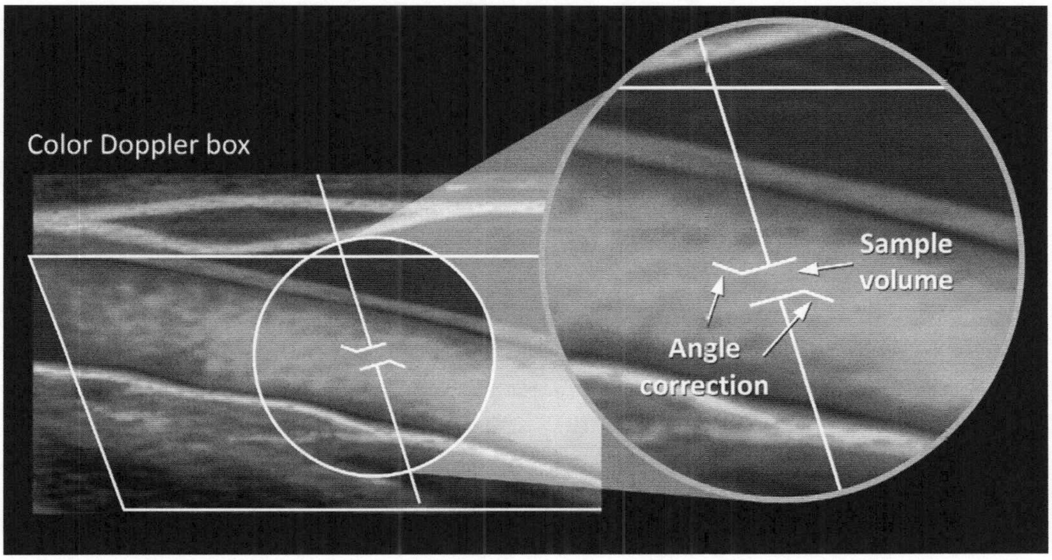

Pulse Repetition Frequency

Pulse repetition frequency (PRF) is the number of ultrasonic pulses occurring in one second. This value is usually expressed in kilohertz (kHz). Doppler ultrasound scanners use pulsed wave systems. The major advantages of using a pulsed wave system is that it allows measurement of depth and that the sample volume can be adjusted by the operator. For these reasons, pulsed wave ultrasound is used to provide data for color flow images. A limitation of pulsed wave ultrasound is that the maximum Doppler frequency that can be accurately measured (without aliasing) is only one-half of the pulse repetition frequency.

Sources of Artifacts

Sources of artifacts:

- Acoustic interactions within tissues
- Instrumental factors (failures)
- Implanted devices
- Operator induced

Most tissue artifacts are well understood and taken into account for diagnoses.

Refraction Artifacts and Reverberation Artifacts

Refraction is ultrasound beam bending that occurs when the incident beam is not perpendicular to the target structure. It commonly occurs where bone meets soft tissue. Refraction may produce images that are not viewed in their correct positions on the ultrasound monitor. This may result in an inability to accurately measure characteristics such as length or depth. Reverberation occurs when the ultrasound beam reflects off of tissues that have different levels of acoustic impedance (resistance to vibration). Reverberations appear as equally spaced, bright rings that decrease in brightness as the transducer face moves away.

Ring-Down Artifact and Comet-Tail Artifact

A ring-down artifact is indicative of abdominal gas pockets such as those seen in pneumobilia (the presence of gas in the biliary ducts). It appears as a solid streak (or parallel bands) radiating away from the gas pocket itself.

The comet-tail artifact appears as multiple, small, white streaks running parallel to the target structure. It is caused by the reflection of the ultrasound beam off of small, spherical, reflective objects (such as gas bubbles or stones).

Enhancement and Shadowing Artifacts

Clinicians may use ultrasound artifacts as a tool to increase diagnostic confidence. For example, if a structure is fluid filled, posterior enhancement should be visualized posterior to the cyst. Anything that is filled with fluid will appear anechoic because it has a lower attenuation rate. The surrounding tissue that is below anything that is fluid filled will appear brighter and is known as an enhancement artifact. While evaluating the ovaries, the enhancement artifact helps clinicians discern that the structure is fluid filled. Shadowing is the opposite of an enhancement artifact; this is a hypoechoic area posterior to a highly attenuating structure. This hypoechoic area prevents users from being able to see any underlying anatomy to these objects, but it provides clues of stones or calcifications. Sonographers may visualize small calcifications within the ovary, artery, or even within blood vessels.

Edge Shadowing

When a sonographer visualizes a shadow protruding from the edge of a curved structure that is parallel to the axis of the ultrasound beam, it may be referred to as an edge shadow. These artifacts are portrayed as thin, hypoechoic structures that may actually prevent a user from visualizing underlying anatomical structures. These artifacts are created from a decrease in intensity as a sound beam refracts and diverges at the same time after making contact with a curved reflector. Refraction will take place when the propagation speeds are different in the presence of oblique incidence. These artifacts are often seen when performing an ultrasound of a cyst or during a testicular scan. Other examples may include a transverse image of the gallbladder or fetal head due to the curvature of these structures.

Mirror Artifact

A mirror artifact will always be visualized at a depth greater than that of the actual structure being imaged. It is known as a mirror artifact because a very strong reflector tends to redirect the sound waves as it strikes the mirror. This mirror will appear between the actual object being imaged and the second copy of the structure. The second copy will be equidistant from the reflector as the object, but it will be at a greater depth. This artifact can appear not only in grayscale imaging, but also during color Doppler interrogation. In this case, a second vessel may appear deeper than the actual vessel, but it is actually a mirror artifact. When imaging the abdomen, a common mirror imaging artifact visualized is lung tissue on either side of the diaphragm, which is seen as a bright reflector.

Cleaning Up Low-Level Reflections in the Near Field of a Well-Distended Urinary Bladder

When a sonographer notices low-level reflections within the near field of a well-distended urinary bladder and would like to clean them up, he or she may do so using the reject control on the ultrasound system. On some machines, this may be known as rejection, threshold, or suppression, and it can be used to exclude weakened echoes from appearing on the ultrasound screen. Electronic noise produces low-level reflections, so the reject control can be used to reduce this noise. Because every echo must have a set minimum amplitude in order to be displayed, this control determines what that value is so that the signals are not processed, thus eliminating the noise.

Artifacts Encountered When Color Doppler Imaging Is Used

Doppler gain artifacts must be corrected so that data are not lost or misinterpreted. In order to get the entire vessel to fill in properly, one of the first steps that the sonographer can perform after turning on color flow is to adjust the pulse repetition frequency (PRF), which is often referred to as the color scale when color Doppler is activated. In arteries, the blood is flowing rapidly, so the ultrasound user would want to increase the PRF. This raises the Nyquist limit of the machine, which will help avoid aliasing. Aliasing can occur in color Doppler imaging and will appear as a variety of colors within the lumen of the blood vessel. The next step the sonographer may take is to increase the color gain if the vessel is not completely filled with color. Color Doppler is often used during venous duplex exams of the extremities. In this example, the sonographer is trying to optimize color flow in the smaller vessels of a patient's lower leg. If color flow is not immediately visualized after turning on color Doppler, the sonographer should adjust the PRF, otherwise known as the color scale.

Aliasing Artifact and Corrective Measures to Take When Using Spectral Doppler

Spectral analysis is a tool that identifies every velocity obtained within the signal that is reflected. However, when there are aliasing errors in the spectral waveform, the interpreting physician may mistake the data as true information, which could lead to a misdiagnosis. Aliasing is considered an artifact that demonstrates an error in imaging because the waveform tends to wrap around the baseline. There are many steps that can be taken to eliminate signals that display aliasing. The first step a sonographer should try is to adjust the pulse repetition frequency (PRF) (velocity scale). In arteries, the blood flow is moving rapidly so increasing the PRF may help unwrap the spectral display. This step increases the Nyquist limit, which is also known as the aliasing frequency and is equal to half of the PRF. If this alone does not take care of aliasing, the baseline may be adjusted accordingly. Another helpful tip to eliminate aliasing is to switch to a lower frequency transducer or even find a window that is at a shallower location. The angle of incidence could also be increased to help eliminate aliasing. If that still doesn't work, then the user could switch to continuous-wave Doppler.

Differentiating Between Flow Reversal and Aliasing During an Exam Using Color Doppler

It is important for sonographers to realize that aliasing can occur not only with spectral Doppler analysis, but also with color flow Doppler. The user must be able to discern between aliasing and the reversal of flow (bidirectional flow). In order to determine if aliasing is present, the user must pay close attention to the color map located on the side of the image. If the colors on the map tend to wrap from the top around the outside and to the bottom of the map, then users may assume that aliasing is present. If the colors on the middle of the color map communicate with each other, then bidirectional flow is present. The best step that an ultrasound user can take in order to remove an aliasing artifact from a color Doppler exam is to increase the level of the velocity scale.

Artifacts Visualized Due to Patient Motion When Using Power Doppler

A disadvantage of power Doppler imaging (PDI) is that the study may suffer because of flash artifact. Flash artifact occurs not because of the motion of the red blood cells, but rather it is a burst of color visualized when there is motion taking place outside of the blood vessels. Often, this motion is caused by patient motion. Examples of patient motion may be that the patient is actually moving on the exam table, but it may also be involuntary motion such as movement of the heart or lungs during respiration. Flash artifact may also appear because of motion caused by the transducer as the sonographer is moving it on the patient or even motion caused from the pressure that the transducer places on soft-tissue structures. Flash artifact may appear as a randomized burst of color, occurring outside of the vessels.

Role of Intermittent Sampling in Pulsed-Wave Doppler Aliasing Artifacts

Aliasing is common during pulsed-wave Doppler exams due to intermittent sampling. Intermittent sampling occurs if the Doppler frequency is not evaluated correctly. When the Doppler frequency is larger than the Nyquist limit, which is equal to half of the pulse repetition frequency (PRF), then aliasing will take place. Aliasing is when the blood flow direction is incorrectly portrayed either above or below the baseline; it will wind around the entire spectral window and appear to move in the opposite direction. Aliasing can also arise when color flow Doppler is being used, so ultrasound users should be able to identify if it is present. Aliasing will never occur with continuous-wave Doppler because it can only be the result of pulsed ultrasound technology.

Aliasing in Color Doppler Exams

Color Doppler uses grayscale imaging to locate the anatomical structures, and when activated, a color box will be layered on top of the B-mode image. This information includes data about the mean velocity of blood moving through various structures instead of peak velocity as measured by pulsed-wave and continuous-wave Doppler. Color Doppler does provide information regarding the direction of blood flow, and it is prone to aliasing. Ultrasound users should be able to tell the difference between color Doppler that is aliasing and flow that is moving in the reverse direction. The operator must pay close attention to the color map displayed on the screen. Just as pulsed-wave Doppler that is aliasing tends to wrap around the spectral window, color Doppler that is aliasing winds around the top of the color box around to the bottom.

Adjusting the Baseline to Eliminate Aliasing

During a spectral display, the system can document flow that is moving in opposite directions. Flow that is visualized above the baseline demonstrates flow that is moving toward the transducer. Flow below the baseline signifies blood flow traveling away from the transducer. If the user notices that flow is wrapping around the baseline, this is an aliasing artifact. Sonographers can take many steps to eliminate aliasing. One such corrective measure that can be done is to adjust the baseline. If the flow is above the baseline but aliasing occurs, the user can move the baseline lower so that the entire waveform is going in one direction. This allows for extremely high velocity flow to be shown moving in the correct direction and still allows for an accurate measurement.

Correcting an Aliasing Artifact During a Carotid Duplex Exam Imaged at 35 Degrees with a 10 MHz Transducer

Spectral Doppler waveforms can provide clinicians with a lot of insight pertaining to blood flowing throughout the body. Blood does not necessarily travel in the same speed or direction, even within the same blood vessel. Spectral analysis is a tool that identifies every velocity obtained within the signal that is reflected. However, when there are aliasing errors in the spectral waveform, the interpreting physician may mistake that data as true information. This could lead to a misdiagnosis. In this example, a 10 MHz transducer is creating an aliasing artifact so the sonographer may try to reduce the transducer's Doppler frequency. The PRF scale could also be increased to raise the Nyquist limit, and the baseline could be moved down. If that doesn't work, the user could increase the angle of incidence or switch to continuous-wave Doppler.

Clinical Care, Practice, and Quality Assurance

Assessment of Patient During Ultrasound

The ultrasound technician must understand how to assess a patient during an ultrasound examination. The technician should look at the color of the patient and the way the patient is breathing. The technician should be able to take a pulse, assess heart rate and respiratory rate, call for assistance in the case of an emergency, and tell how the patient is tolerating the procedure. If a patient is on a cardiac monitor, the technician should be familiar with the normal way the heart rate appears on the monitor screen and be able to pick up on changes a patient may be experiencing during the procedure. The technician should have a basic understanding that an adult heart rate is normally between 60-100 beats per minute and that a child's rate can be between 100-120 beats per minute. An infant or neonate can have a heart rate even higher. Understanding normal heart and respiratory rates helps the sonographer recognize when a patient is experiencing distress.

Clinical Data

Indications

Polycystic Renal Disease

Renal cystic disease consists of inflammatory or necrotic cysts. The most common of these is inherited polycystic renal disease (or PRD). PRD is marked by the formation of fluid-filled cysts in the kidney tubules. These cysts compress functioning kidney tissue, eventually replacing it. In the more common type (autosomal dominant PRD), almost half of the patients develop chronic kidney failure between the ages of 40 and 60. The rare form (autosomal recessive PRD) causes kidney failure in early childhood. In most cases of renal cystic disease both kidneys typically show enlargement. Patients may experience back (or flank) pain, red blood cells in the urine (hematuria), white blood cells (leukocytes) in the urine, and excess protein in the urine (proteinuria).

Kidney Stones

Kidney stones (renal calculi) are solid crystals made up of dissolved minerals that occur in urine. They are typically found inside the kidneys or ureters. The size of the stone can be as large as a golf ball. Tiny kidney stones usually leave the body in the urine stream unnoticed. The larger stones can cause an obstruction of a ureter. This in turn causes the ureter to swell with urine and causes moderate to severe pain. The pain is most commonly felt in the back (flank), lower abdomen, and groin. The most common composition of kidney stones is calcium oxalate. Clinical symptoms of kidney stones include intermittent back (flank) pain, vomiting, red blood cells in the urine (hematuria), infection, and an elevated white blood cell (leukocyte) count.

Renal Inflammation

Inflammation of the kidneys (nephritis) is the primary characteristic of several kidney diseases. In the most common type, glomerulonephritis (also known as Bright's disease), the glomerulus (the filtering part of the kidney) becomes inflamed and scarred. The kidneys slowly lose their ability to remove wastes and excess water from the blood to make urine. Diseases such as diabetes and lupus can cause glomerulonephritis. The disease may be acute or chronic in nature. Abscesses and bacterial infections are also common causes of nephritis. Typical symptoms include back (or flank) pain, fever, elevated white blood cell (leukocyte) count, and pus in the urine (pyuria). In some cases, there is also an increase in blood urea nitrogen (BUN), albumen, and total plasma protein levels.

Symptoms, Clinical Correlation, and Associated Complications for Liver Diseases

Liver disease may originate in a number of areas. Hepatitis (liver inflammation) is usually caused by viral infection, exposure to toxins (including alcohol and drugs), or autoimmune factors. Portal hypertension and metabolic diseases also cause many liver problems. The liver can be injured by benign and malignant tumors (including cysts). The liver may also become involved in a number of systemic conditions, including autoimmune disorders, infections, and heart failure. Liver disease usually shows similar clinical manifestations. Initially, symptoms are typically mild. This sturdy and resilient organ can compensate for a surprising amount of damage. Eventually evidence of liver failure occurs; this is characterized by a marked decline in liver functions and the development of swelling (due to fluid retention) and portal hypertension. Additional signs of liver disease include:

- Jaundice (hyperbilirubinemia)
- Cirrhosis (irreversible fibrosis and scarring)
- Hepatocellular carcinoma (primary malignant cancer of the liver)
- Hepatic failure (severe decline in all liver functions).

Symptoms, Clinical Correlation, and Complications for Pancreas Diseases

The two most common symptomatic diseases of the pancreas are pancreatitis (inflammation of the pancreas) and pancreatic cancer.

Following are the most common symptoms of pancreatitis:

- Nausea and/or vomiting.
- A feeling of a fast pulse or sustained heart rate increase.
- A general feeling of illness.
- The presence of a fever.
- The presence of swelling in the upper abdomen.
- A build-up of fluid in the abdominal cavity (ascites).
- Low (or dropping) blood pressure readings.
- In acute pancreatitis there is usually moderate to severe pain in the upper abdomen.

Following are the most common symptoms of pancreatic cancer:

- Sustained pain in the upper abdomen.
- A loss of appetite.
- A rapid loss of weight.
- The presence of jaundice (yellowing of the skin and eyes).
- Chronic indigestion.
- Nausea and/or vomiting.

Laboratory Tests

Urinalysis

Urinalysis is useful for detecting kidney function problems. The presence of red blood cells (hematuria) or pus (pyuria) in the urine can indicate an infection of the urinary tract.

pH of Urine Test

The filtrate of blood plasma (filtered through the glomerulus within the kidney) is usually acidified by renal tubules and collecting ducts from a pH of seven (neutral) to about six (slightly acidic) in the final urine. However, depending on the acid-base balance, urinary pH may range from a low of four to as high as eight. The formation of kidney stones (calculi) and the presence of bacteria in the urine (bacteriuria) are conditions dependent on urine pH levels. Also, alkaline urine (pH greater than seven) is a symptom of tubular acidosis and chronic renal failure.

Specific Gravity

Specific gravity (a fluid's weight per unit of volume) is dependent on the amount of solids dissolved in the fluid. For urine, specific gravity can be used to determine the kidney's ability to concentrate urine. If a person drinks a large amount of water, the urine will be more dilute (less waste per unit of volume) and its corresponding specific gravity will be lower. Conversely, if a person becomes dehydrated, the urine will become more concentrated (more waste per unit of volume) and their urine's specific gravity will be higher. Diseases that cause renal tubular damage impair the kidney's ability to concentrate urine. Examples of these diseases include; renal failure, glomerular nephritis (caused by inflammation of the internal kidney structures (glomeruli)), and pyelonephritis (an infection of the kidney and the ducts that carry urine).

Hemoglobin

Hemoglobin in the urine is indicative of damage or death of the body's red blood cells (erythrocytes). If left untreated, this condition can be very damaging to the kidneys and lead to acute renal failure.

Protein

When the internal kidney structures (glomeruli) become damaged, albumen and other proteins may be filtered from the bloodstream in abnormally high amounts. This leads to a shortage of proteins in the blood and higher than normal levels of proteins in the urine (albuminuria). Patients with either benign or malignant kidney tumors, kidney stones (calculi), chronic infections or pyelonephritis (an infection of the kidney and the ducts that carry urine) may be affected by this condition.

Creatinine

Creatinine is a waste molecule that is generated from muscle metabolism. It is produced from creatine, a molecule used for energy production in muscles. Creatinine is transported through the bloodstream to the kidneys. The kidneys filter out most of the creatinine and eliminate it from the body in the urine. The kidneys maintain blood creatinine levels in a normal range. Creatinine has been found to be a fairly reliable indicator of kidney function. As the kidneys become impaired the creatinine level in the blood will rise. This is known as poor creatinine clearance. Abnormally high blood levels of creatinine thus warn of possible malfunction or failure of the kidneys, in many cases even before a patient reports any symptoms. It is for this reason that standard blood and urine tests routinely check for the amount of creatinine.

Blood in Urine Test

An early sign of renal disease is the presence of blood in the urine. A large amount of red blood cells in the urine may be due to blunt trauma to the kidney, kidney stones (calculi), or pyelonephritis (an infection of the kidney and the ducts that carry urine). Alternatively, the condition may be caused by glomerular or vascular inflammation. The presence of white blood cells (leukocytes) in the urine may be due to inflammation, infection, or tissue death (necrosis) anywhere in the urinary tract.

Hematocrit Test

The blood hematocrit ratio is the ratio of plasma to packed cell volume in the blood. Decreased hematocrit is associated with acute bleeding caused by disease or blunt trauma.

Blood Urea Nitrogen Test

The blood urea nitrogen (BUN) test measures the amount of nitrogen in your blood that comes from urea (a waste product produced by the liver when proteins are broken down). Urea is eliminated from the body in the urine. The BUN test is performed to evaluate how well the kidneys are functioning. If the kidneys are unable to remove urea from the blood, the patient's BUN level increases. Heart failure, dehydration, or a diet high in protein (example: the Atkins diet) can increase the BUN level. BUN levels decrease when there is impairment in liver function (usually due to physical damage or disease). This is because urea is produced in the liver. A decreased BUN level also can occur normally in the second or third trimester of pregnancy.

Diagnostic Liver Function Blood Tests

These diagnostic blood tests are used as a first course to determine the cause of potential liver-related problems in the patient. Some usual symptoms include; jaundice, dark urine, light or black colored feces, nausea/vomiting (including blood), swelling/pain in the abdomen, and unusual weight change. Higher elevations of AST and ALT can be signs of the death and damage of liver cells. This may be the result of acute and chronic diseases of the liver such as hepatitis and cirrhosis. Higher elevations of Alk Phos and bilirubin can indicate blockage of the bile ducts. This may be the result of gallstones or a structural tissue injury within the liver. Lower levels of albumin in the blood (and a longer PT time) are indicative of a severe problem with the liver's metabolic ability.

Lactic Acid Dehydrogenase Test

The presence of elevated levels of lactic acid dehydrogenase (LDH) results from the death or damage of cells in various tissues of the body (such as the heart, kidneys, or liver). The role of LDH is to convert lactic acid (produced by muscle tissue during stress) into pyruvic acid (that is necessary to produce energy within the cells). LDH isoenzymes can be used to isolate the specific tissue that has been affected.

Alkaline Phosphatase Test

The presence of highly elevated alkaline phosphatase (Alk Phos or ALP) levels indicates a blockage of the bile ducts. Levels of ALP are also high in patients with liver or bone cancer. ALP isoenzymes can also be used to isolate their source (such as the liver or bones).

Aspartate Aminotransferase or Serum Glutamic Oxaloacetic Transaminase Test

Aspartate aminotransferase (AST) (also called Serum glutamic oxaloacetic transaminase (SGOT)) is an enzyme primarily associated with liver and heart cells. Its level in the blood rises in direct proportion to the number of dead or damaged cells in these organs. Liver diseases such as acute hepatitis and cirrhosis cause sustained elevations of this enzyme in the blood.

Alanine Aminotransferase Test

Alanine aminotransferase (ALT) is an enzyme (more sensitive to liver cells than AST) that is released into the blood when these cells die or are damaged. The level is in proportion to the number of dead or damaged cells (primarily in the liver). The AST and ALT tests may be performed at the same time to gain additional information. The ratio of AST to ALT may be used as an indicator as to whether the liver (or another organ) has been mostly affected.

Prothrombin Time

Prothrombin time (PT) is a test designed to measure the length of time it takes for blood to clot. It is typically used to determine bleeding problems. Prothrombin (factor II) is one of the clotting factors produced by the liver. The ability for the liver to produce prothrombin is determined by the availability of vitamin K. An increase in PT indicates damage to the liver cells (typically caused by disease).

Albumin and Globulins

The blood levels of albumin and globulins are measured to determine liver function. Solely produced by the liver, albumin is the major blood protein used by the body (the remainder are globulins). Many drugs, fats, hormones and toxins are bound to albumin in the bloodstream and carried to the liver for processing to water-soluble forms. A low blood level of albumin indicates a significant impairment of the liver (usually caused by cirrhosis).

Indirect Bilirubin, Direct Bilirubin, and Total Bilirubin

Bilirubin is the major bile pigment that is produced when hemoglobin is broken down in the blood. The resulting indirect (or unconjugated) bilirubin is carried to the liver (by albumin) to be processed. Indirect bilirubin is fat-soluble and must be converted (by the liver) to a water-soluble form (called direct or conjugated bilirubin) in order to be eliminated from the body. Normally, only a low level of bilirubin exists in the blood. When the liver is damaged or unable to properly process indirect bilirubin, the total bilirubin level (indirect bilirubin plus direct bilirubin) increases in the bloodstream. When the total bilirubin builds to a high level, a yellowing of the skin and eyes (called jaundice) is typically observable in the patient. In adults, high blood levels of bilirubin are typically due to gallstones or liver diseases (such as cirrhosis or hepatitis).

Lab Tests to Determine Pancreatic Insufficiency

The following lab tests are used to diagnose pancreatic (exocrine function) insufficiency:

- Fecal fat test: Pancreatic sourced enzymes break down dietary fats so that they may be absorbed by the intestinal wall of the small intestine. If the pancreas cannot supply the precursors to these necessary enzymes, the body has difficulty absorbing dietary fat and it is excreted in the patient's feces. This quantitative test measures the amount of fat expelled in the feces and compares it a normal value.
- Trypsin test: Trypsin is a pancreatic-sourced enzyme that breaks down dietary protein (into peptides) so that it may be absorbed by the intestinal wall of the small intestine. If the pancreas cannot supply the precursors to these necessary enzymes, the body has difficulty absorbing protein. The absence of trypsin in a patient's feces indicates that the pancreas is not functioning normally.

The following lab tests are used to determine pancreatic (endocrine function) insufficiency:

- Blood sugar (glucose) levels: The pancreas produces both insulin and glucagon that are used by the body to control blood levels of glucose. If the pancreas does not produce enough insulin, blood sugar levels rise to abnormally high levels resulting in hyperglycemia. If the pancreas produces too much insulin (hyperinsulinemia), abnormally low blood sugar levels are possible resulting in hypoglycemia.

- Insulin levels also affect liver function, which plays a key role in maintaining normal blood sugar levels. After eating (when insulin levels are elevated) the liver stores excess glucose in the form of glycogen. Throughout the day (when insulin levels decrease) the liver breaks down glycogen and releases the stored glucose into the bloodstream. This keeps blood sugar levels within a narrow and normal range.

Prostate Specific Antigen Lab Test

The PSA test measures the blood level of prostate specific antigen (PSA). PSA is a reproductive enzyme produced by the prostate that helps sperm move through the female's cervix. Generally, PSA levels less than 4 ng/ml (nanograms per milliliter) are viewed as normal for men less than fifty years of age. The PSA level tends to rise naturally with age, and some labs raise the level considered normal accordingly. In any case, PSA levels higher than ten may be associated with prostate cancer. Other causes of abnormally high PSA levels are benign prostatic hyperplasia (BPH) and infection of the prostate (prostatitis).

Gallbladder and Biliary Tests

The following liver function tests are used to diagnose diseases of the gallbladder and biliary tree:

- Lactate dehydrogenase (LDH). LDH is an enzyme that is present in many body tissues, especially the heart, liver, kidney, skeletal muscle, brain, blood cells, and lungs. When these tissues are damaged, LDH is released to the blood.
- Alk Phos (alkaline phosphatase) and GGT (gamma-glutamyltranspeptidase). Alk Phos and GGT bloodstream levels are elevated in a number of disorders that affect the drainage of bile (such as a gallstone, cyst or tumor blocking the common bile duct). Since alkaline phosphatase is also found in other organs, GGT is utilized as a confirmatory test to be sure that the elevation of alkaline phosphatase is indeed coming from the liver or the biliary tree.
- Serum glutamic oxaloacetic transaminase (SGOT) or aspartate aminotransferase (AST). This is an enzyme that is normally present in liver and heart cells. It is released into the blood when there is damage to the heart (such as occurs with a heart attack) or to the liver (such as occurs with cirrhosis).
- Serum glutamic pyruvic transaminase (SGPT) or alanine aminotransferase (ALT). Similar to SGOT, this is another enzyme that is released to the blood when heart or liver cells are damaged. This enzyme is more specific to liver cell damage than SGOT.

The blood levels of these enzymes rise and then fall back to normal for acute disorders and remains elevated for chronic disorders.

Correlating Ultrasound Findings with Other Imaging Modalities

Ultrasound is often the first modality that is used to evaluate patients that present with pain, swelling, palpable masses, or abnormal lab values. Sonographers should always determine if the patient has had prior imaging exams pertaining to this issue before starting the exam so that a comparison can be made. Often, the patient may recall having an exam but may be confused as to which exam was performed. It is also important for other technologists (computed tomography [CT], magnetic resonance imaging, nuclear medicine) to do the same and compare any imaging studies to prior ultrasounds. Along with the actual exam, it is important for any technologist to carefully read any report, especially in cases where a follow-up has been indicated. For example, if a patient has three nodules that were previously visualized in the liver on a CT of the abdomen, the sonographer must make sure that all three lesions are properly documented. Some systems allow the ultrasound operator to upload a prior CT exam into their ultrasound system so that the CT image is next to the live ultrasound exam so the radiologist knows that the information obtained is on the correct lesion.

Spatial Compounding

Spatial compounding is the technology that acquires data from multiple imaging angles and combines them into one image. These frames are generated by one stationary transducer, and then the frames are processed into one image. Steering is used from not only the center of the ultrasound beam, but also from the right and left sides of the transducer. Resolution is greatly improved when spatial compounding is used because more data are obtained and combined. A higher quality of spatial compounding is generated, of course, with a higher number of frame rates. Spatial compounding will degrade temporal resolution, however, because when more processing is required, the frame rate tends to slow down. This is a technology that is useful to reduce speckle and shadowing artifacts. It is useful in exams such as musculoskeletal, thyroid, vascular, and breast ultrasounds.

Picture Archiving and Communications System

The picture archiving and communications system (PACS) allows users of digital imaging to electronically share and archive images so that they can be viewed on a network. Clinicians and other medical personnel can also access diagnostic imaging reports because they can be stored on PACS. PACS has been used to replace film for facilities that have converted to digital imaging systems. This not only saves storage space for the film and chemicals used to process film within imaging departments, but it also allows more than one user to visualize studies at the same time as well as grants instantaneous access to the stored images. If a patient comes into the emergency department (ED) with an abdominal aortic aneurysm, not only can an ED physician view the images, but a surgeon can also see the images in the operating room. Over time, film studies tend to deteriorate, and this will not occur with studies that are archived with PACS.

Digital Imaging and Computers in Medicine

Digital Imaging and Computers in Medicine (DICOM) can be thought of as the link between the ultrasound machine (or any other digital imaging system) and the PACS system. DICOM allows for the integration of the networks, printing devices, workstations, and PACS that may have been purchased (often from multiple vendors). These protocols allow the ultrasound machine to send the images to the PACS network for archiving purposes. In contrast to JPEG images, DICOM images are extremely large, and one cannot just load these images onto their computer. DICOM data are not recognized by Windows, so users cannot just double-click on an image to load it. A DICOM browser is necessary so that the images can be viewed on various computers, workstations, or even a CD.

Standards and Guidelines

Importance of Obtaining Written Consent and Labs Prior to Ultrasound

Ultrasound operators must be certain to obtain a consent form from every patient that is scanned (either on paper or electronically). State and federal regulations require proof of this record, and proper documentation demonstrates that the patient was provided a sufficient amount of information about the exam to be performed. The written consent form is not only for the procedural steps of the exam, but that the benefits, any associated risks, and other options for treatment were communicated to the patient. Patients should always speak to the physician performing the exam to make sure that all of his or her questions or concerns are addressed. It is, of course, the patient's prerogative to opt out of any procedure whether it is prior to or during an exam. Lab values should always be obtained prior to any procedure because these results may offer the provider ample amounts of data pertaining to the patient's health. For example, it is important to know that the patient's liver or kidneys are functioning normally or if their blood clots properly.

ALARA Principle

The ALARA, or "as low as reasonably achievable," principle stresses the use of the lowest reasonable energy used to achieve the result of a clear image. It recognizes that there are bio-effects of ultrasound and patient safety is important. The Food and Drug Administration regulates ultrasound instruments and the application, intensities, and thermal and mechanical indexes to be used. The American Institute of Ultrasound in Medicine recommends the safe and prudent use of sound waves in the clinical arena and only when needed. Keep exposure to a minimum. Achieve the information with as little energy exposure to the client as possible and still get an appropriate image for diagnostic result. Acoustic exposure is the energy the patient receives during a scan. The intensity varies across the beam. It is highest at the center and least intense at the periphery. The lowest intensity would be for gray-scale imaging and the most intense would be color Doppler. Pulse-wave Doppler is more intense than continuous-wave Doppler.

Regular Duties Regardless of Examination Type Performed

The technician must do routine quality assurance tests to make certain the ultrasound lab is being run efficiently. They must clean and prepare all transducers after each examination and be prepared for the next patient. Someone in the department is responsible for ordering equipment and supplies and someone is responsible for checking the orders for the next day, scheduling patients, and preparing those patients for their exams. A technician is responsible for recording and generating images, storing those images or transmitting them to the appropriate physicians, and for archiving all of the images for future reference. There is someone responsible for clean linen in the department, having gels and extra supplies in each ultrasound room, and for providing the patient with gowns, towels, and sterile trays for possible procedures each day.

Role of Sonographer During Ultrasound Procedure

The sonographer must first review the physician order and verify the scan that is to be done. It is also helpful to review other tests that have been conducted. The sonographer should identify himself or herself to the patient and address the patient by name. Explain the examination to the family and to the patient. Obtain a brief medical history, especially involving allergies and latex sensitivity. Verify the patient name, date, birth date, or medical record number and make certain the numbers are correct on the imaging screen. Select the proper transducer frequency and use the one limiting the acoustic output in compliance with the ALARA, or "as low as reasonably achievable," principle. Maintain the privacy of the patient and protect his or her privacy. Address the patient's concerns regarding the examination. Explain the expected time of reading and when the patient can expect to get the results from the physician.

When to Call a Physician

A physician should be contacted when the ultrasound findings would indicate an immediate intervention. Urgent findings would include an ectopic pregnancy, abruptio placentae, or a leaking aneurysm. These are examples of the need for emergent surgical intervention. Fetal death, fetal anomalies, and abnormal fetal heart rate are examples of pathology that may need an intervention and should not wait for a dictated report to be sent to an office; calling the physician at the completion of the examination is the standard. Other serious conditions that should be phoned to the physician include: unexpected neoplastic masses; large hematomas; renal artery occlusion in kidney transplant patients; obstructed bile ducts; and placenta previa and bleeding.

Patient Preparation for Gallbladder Ultrasound

The patient should fast for 8-12 hours before a scan to offer a better window for the imaging. It allows for less air in the stomach and gives room for water if needed to get a clearer image. Use a transducer with a high frequency and set the focal zone to the back wall of the gallbladder where stones collect. The frequency must be strong enough to go through the entire organ but may be changed when scanning the liver to avoid subtle shadowing. Harmonic imaging may help clear artifacts. Start with positioning the patient in a supine position. It is also advisable to get left lateral decubitus views, oblique, and prone views so not to miss scanning a gallbladder stone. The upright position is an awkward position for the patient but may be helpful if the liver is small or high in the quadrant. A standing position for this upright scan is often better and offers an acoustic window which enhances the view of the gallbladder.

Positioning for Basic Ultrasound Exams

The sonographer progresses through very extensive training to learn techniques and positioning of both the patient, the transducers, and the sound beams when doing an ultrasound examination. The patient must be correctly positioned for each individual examination for the best acoustic window and to gain the best images of a specific organ or tissue. There are common positions for routine scans. The supine or dorsal recumbent position is the position where the patient lies on his or her back looking straight up. Sometimes a pillow can be placed under the knees or the head for comfort. This is used to examine the abdomen, ribs, and pelvis. A side-lying position, known as the lateral position, may allow the patient to elevate the dependent arm above the head. One leg is straight and one bent for comfort and support. The prone position is lying on the abdomen with arms flexed at each side. The feet may extend off the examination table and a small pillow may be used for comfort for the head.

Orientation of a Sagittal Scan Sonogram

The sagittal (or longitudinal) scanning plane is that which runs from the head to the foot and divides the patient into right and left halves. Some examples of structures that are seen in the sagittal plane are the uterus and cervix. The correct orientation of a sagittal scan sonogram is as follows:

- Posterior is at the bottom of the sonogram
- For a sagittal scan through the pancreas and aorta, the direction of the patient's feet is on the right side of the sonogram
- For a sagittal scan in the right breast, the direction of the patient's head is on the left side of the sonogram.

Standard Right and Left Upper Quadrant Abdominal Examination

The longitudinal (sagittal) views should be used with the left and right upper quadrants. The scan should include the aorta and the distal aorta especially in patients over the age of 55. The scan should include the inferior vena cava, the main lobar fissure, and the gallbladder. Always include the head of the pancreas, the right and left kidneys, and the side aspect of the liver so the diaphragm and pleural spaces can be seen. Scans should include images of the spleen, the adrenal glands, and any abnormalities seen. Color Doppler can be used to view the main portal vein which will point out blood flow. Transverse views can include the levels of the portal veins, the common duct, the hepatic artery, and the neck, body, and fundus of the gallbladder, as well as the pancreatic region.

Orientation of a Transverse Scan Sonogram

Transverse scanning is used to image structures that lie transversely (sideways) within the body (such as the pancreas). The transverse plane divides the body into upper and lower portions and extends from side to side. The correct orientation of a transverse scan sonogram is as follows:

- For a transverse scan through the left thyroid, the patient's right side is on the left of the sonogram
- For a transverse scan of the gallbladder, the patient's left side is on the right of the sonogram
- For a transverse scan of the left kidney, the top of the sonogram represents the anterior

Safety Considerations While Performing Ultrasound

Technicians should use good body mechanics to protect themselves from injury. The sonographer must understand and follow the policies when a patient is in isolation which may include wearing a gown, gloves, or mask when performing an ultrasound on an infected patient. The sonographer should be aware of oxygen safety, electrical safety, and the use of proper electrical cords when performing an ultrasound. The ultrasound equipment should be in safe working order and care should be taken with the plugs to avoid tripping over them, having a patient trip, or having the cords near any water spill. The sonographer should always be aware of the location of the fire alarms, the cardiac arrest alarm, and how to call for help quickly in the case of a medical emergency during an ultrasound examination. The sonographer should be aware of proper positioning and body mechanics when moving and transferring a patient from chair to examination table.

General Safety Protocols

Infection-Control Procedures

The technician must practice good hand-washing techniques from patient to patient. Masks may be worn for suspected fluid splatter as well as gowns or goggles. Disposal of fluid soaked linen, garbage, or specimens must be handled carefully and following the institution's policies. The sonographer may need to follow specific isolation precautions depending on the patient and the diagnosis. The scanning probe and transducers must be cleansed with appropriate cleaners; taking care to clean the cords, cable, and head of the transducer. It is usually advised to use a partial bleach solution to clean equipment and carts, counters, and sinks after completion of the examination and when the patient has left. The technician is responsible for knowing how to provide sterile techniques when appropriate.

Precautions

The various types of precautions are described below:

- Standard precautions are guidelines that should be followed to prevent exposure to blood or body fluids from all patients. These provide standards for protective gear to be worn, disposable of sharps, cleaning body fluid spills, and isolation room guidelines.
- Transmission-based precautions are used when a specific disease state is known. They are guidelines followed to prevent transmission of this disease. An example of this would be the isolation room requirements and protective gear used when caring for patients with tuberculosis.
- Airborne precautions outline the procedures to prevent transmission of diseases which are transmitted through the air. This includes any special masks that should be worn. An example of this is chicken pox (Varicella virus).
- Droplet precautions outline what guidelines should be followed to prevent transmission of diseases which are transmitted by exposure to respiratory droplets. An example of this is tuberculosis.
- Contact precautions are followed when caring for patients who have diseases that are transmitted through contact with the individual. An example of this is a MRSA skin infection.

Staphylococci Bacteria

Staphylococci bacteria are a very common cause of surgical site infections and have become more difficult to treat. *Staphylococcus epidermidis* is usually not treatable with methicillin, as well as some other common antibiotics. This can become an extremely dangerous infection if it is not treated with appropriate antibiotic therapy. Staphylococci bacteria are very common and many people, especially health care workers, can be colonized with the bacteria. This provides a ready source of bacteria available to infect patients. Most patients are infected through contaminated materials within the hospital or by direct transmission from health care workers. This particular type of bacteria is very resilient, even to standard cleaning products, so extra precaution should be given toward preventing infection in the patient through direct transmission. The most effective means of preventing transmission of organisms is through thorough hand washing before and after contact with a patient. Observing proper Universal Precaution standards also helps to prevent transmission of infectious agents.

Streptococci Bacteria

Streptococci bacteria are common causes of infection. These are responsible for common bacterial respiratory infections in adults, ear infections in children, and severe infections that can be life threatening. There is now an immunization given to young children to help prevent common infections caused by strep bacteria. Group B strep is a bacterium that many people carry without even knowing it. Most pregnant women are tested for colonization with Group B strep before delivery to prevent serious infection in the infant after birth. Group A strep commonly causes skin infections, especially those associated with C-sections and other female reproductive system surgeries. Patients with diabetes and those with depressed immune systems are more susceptible to developing infections by Group A strep. Because strep is so common, antibiotic resistance has developed. The penicillin group of antibiotics is the most effective at treating strep, but has recently been found to be not as effective as in the past because of resistance.

Tuberculosis

Tuberculosis is a serious respiratory illness that has increased in incidence in this country over the past few years. It is seen more frequently in patients who are homeless and those who have decreased immune systems. TB is transmitted through respiratory droplets. Exposure to the disease is evaluated with a PPD skin test. A positive response does not indicate that the person has TB, but rather the person has been exposed to the disease. A positive PPD is usually followed by a chest x-ray to check for the presence of any consolidated areas that may indicate a dormant TB infection. Prophylactic treatment may or may not be done with multiple antibiotics. Patients with TB must wear a specialized TB respiratory mask when being transported through public areas. The TB patient will be placed in a negative-pressure air flow room, on isolation. Strict respiratory/TB precautions should be followed to prevent transmission of the disease to other patients via health care workers.

Standard Hospital Emergency Codes

While no standard system from hospital to hospital yet exists, certain issues may present themselves in hospitals and medical centers. It is important to learn the codes used to identify these situations and to know your role in them, should one occur. Some possibilities are:

- Code Blue – often used to identify a cardiac or respiratory emergency
- Bomb threat – keep the caller on the phone while contacting security
- Child abduction – often identified by Amber Alert or Code Pink. Staff may be assigned to monitor a specific exit
- Combative person – a team may be assembled to present a show of force
- Fire – often identified as Code Red. Know the nearest exit and route.

Code Blue

Code Blue is used in many hospitals and medical centers throughout the country to indicate a medical emergency in which resuscitation is immediately necessary. The most common conditions requiring a Code Blue call are cardiac or respiratory arrest. Code Blue, along with the exact location of the patient, is announced on the hospital intercom system. This is the signal for those personnel assigned to respond to emergencies to arrive on location as quickly as possible. Though the ultrasound technician is not responsible for care of patients, the ultrasound technician should know the facility's procedure for calling a Code Blue, should the technician find a patient in a condition that would warrant Code Blue, or should the patient have a sudden change in condition during an ultrasound. The technician should also be prepared to give the Code Team information regarding what happened just prior to the patient's change in status, including positioning changes or respiratory changes.

Heimlich Maneuver

The Heimlich Maneuver is used to help people who are choking. The maneuver helps to dislodge the food or object that is caught in the airway. The procedure is performed as follows:

- Stand behind the victim, and wrap your arms around him or her.
- Making a fist, position the thumb side of the fist so that it is pressing into the abdomen, above the navel and below the rib cage.
- Holding the fist with the other hand, perform a quick, upward thrust, driving the fist into the upper abdomen.
- Repeat until the object is expelled.
- Heimlich Maneuver training is often included in CPR training programs.

Measurements

Ultrasound Phantoms

A phantom is a structure that contains one or more substitutes for human tissue. It is used to simulate ultrasound interactions in various parts the human body. Phantoms are used to perform numerous tasks on ultrasound equipment such as testing sensitivity, contrast resolution, axial resolution, and lateral resolution. This also includes teaching ultrasound techniques, and servicing the equipment. The most important aspect of a phantom used for ultrasound is that the speed of sound in the test object (phantom) is equal to the speed of sound in the target human tissue.

Measurement Techniques

Various measurement techniques are used during abdominal ultrasound exams to provide physicians with quantitative information. Ultrasound machines have various tools to use that allow ultrasound operators to generate reports so that the information can be presented to the physician in an organized manner. Ultrasound machines also allow users to enter in measurements obtained in prior studies so that the difference can be graphed. Many organs may be measured with calipers to record the length, width, and thickness of a structure. These measurements provide enough information for the machine to also calculate the volume of the organ. Volume can also be calculated with various functions such as an ellipse or even drawing a line around the borders of the organ. Modern systems can also provide information pertaining to the stiffness of the liver to aid in the diagnosis of cirrhosis. Shear-wave elastography is one such technique that provides this quantitative information.

Measurements of Certain Tissues

The measurements of organs, tissues, masses, or cysts should be documented in length and width of each in established normal measurements. The kidney should be measured in the longest length, the perpendicular anteroposterior length, and width. The common bile duct is measured in a sagittal plane and done from where the duct crosses to the main portal vein and hepatic artery. These examples show how the normal accepted anatomy is used to set the standards for measurement. The normal measurements then are used to determine what is abnormal or pathologic. All organs can be measured in length and width. All solid masses or cysts should be measured for size by width and length.

Techniques and Normal Values When Measuring Organs During Abdominal Ultrasounds

Ultrasound systems allow operators to quickly measure organs to provide useful diagnostic information pertaining to the size of the organs. The various lobes of the liver may vary in size and shape, but the left lobe is smaller than the right lobe. The liver is measured from the diaphragm to the inferior tip of the right lobe in a sagittal plane at the midclavicular line. This measurement should not exceed 15.5 cm and is often less than 13 cm. The kidneys should be measured in two planes; they are typically 12 cm long, 5 cm wide, and 2.5 cm thick. The spleen is also measured in order to diagnose splenomegaly. A splenic index is typically calculated and should fall in the 120–480 cm^3 range. If the length of the spleen alone is used as an indicator, it should be less than 13 cm in healthy adults. The pancreas is not typically measured, but it is about 2 cm thick. The pancreatic duct, when seen, should not be more than 2 mm.

Calculating the Volume of a Patient's Spleen

One of the advantages of sonography is quickly being able to measure organs or other anatomical structures within the body. These measurements are useful in the follow-up treatment of many diseases. These measurements can be added to and displayed on a calculations worksheet for the physician that will be interpreting the results. When it is necessary to calculate the volume of an organ, the user will measure the spleen (in this example) in three planes using 2D ultrasound. Volume is displayed in any units of length cubed and is calculated by multiplying the length times the width times the height. Organs are typically measured in centimeters; therefore, the volume is in centimeters cubed (cm^3). Three-dimensional ultrasound is also used to calculate the volume of an organ. This method is actually considered to be superior to measurements obtained on 2D images, but it requires more time to perform.

Sonographic Renal Measurements

A renal ultrasound is a common test ordered when a patient's laboratory results suggest chronic kidney disease. Ultrasound can provide volumetric data of the kidneys as well as measurements of the cortical thickness and images that display the echogenicity. The echogenicity of the kidneys should be compared to the liver and the spleen. Obtaining a renal volume can be a challenge because the kidneys are not elliptical in shape, and it may take experience to get a good volume. This can be difficult when follow-up studies are requested because experience is required, so some clinicians prefer to use the length of the kidney. Another important measurement that may indicate renal disease is cortical thickness. Some studies have shown this as a more accurate indicator of renal function than the length of the kidney. Chronic renal disease will present as kidneys that are smaller than normal with a loss of cortical thickness.

ELASTOGRAPHY

Elastography provides quick and painless measurements of the stiffness of an organ or tissue being interrogated. These measurements are combined with the ultrasound data to create elastograms. B-mode and color Doppler can also be used in conjunction with the elastogram to provide even more information for the clinician. Shear-wave elastography distorts the tissue using the pressure that propagates from the sound wave instead of requiring the sonographer to apply external pressure. Transient elastography of the liver, for example, would require a perpendicular approach from the intercostal region. Once a window is found away from large vessels, the probe button is activated to begin obtaining data. Typically, it is believed that benign structures tend to be softer than their stiffer malignant counterparts. This dynamic technique continues to be evaluated to determine the diagnostic capability it can provide. Elastography offers additional information for breast lesions, liver fibrosis, and musculoskeletal imaging.

MEASUREMENT OF BLOOD FLOW VELOCITY

Spectral analysis is the technique used during pulsed Doppler to provide information pertaining to the various velocities obtained in the blood vessel or organ. Blood doesn't travel in the same direction or speed even when contained in the same sample volume. The spectral analysis window will allow clinicians to examine how the frequency shifts are dispersed within the Doppler signal. Two types of spectral analysis that are used are the fast Fourier transform (FFT) and autocorrelation. FFT is the method used to operate the spectral analysis during pulsed-wave and continuous-wave Doppler. This method can determine if the flow pattern is turbulent or if it is normal (laminar) flow. Autocorrelation is only used during color Doppler, but it is faster than the FFT method. The gate can be moved until it is where the user wants to perform a spectral analysis. The size of the gate can be changed so that it is only within the vessel that is being examined. For example, if one is sampling the carotid artery, but the spectral display is also showing venous flow, the technician will reduce the size of the gate and reposition it so only the artery is being interrogated.

Support

ULTRASOUND GUIDANCE FOR VASCULAR ACCESS PROCEDURES

Ultrasound can be a useful tool when vascular access procedures are required so that clinicians can be sure that the line is placed correctly. The use of ultrasound has proven beneficial because it does not expose the patient to ionizing radiation like fluoroscopy does. Physicians that are trained to perform these procedures with ultrasound guidance can also determine that there is patency of the vessel, the size and depth of the vessel, and tell when the needle is in the best location. It is also possible to visualize if the needle has passed through the posterior wall of a vessel. Surrounding anatomical structures can be visualized within vessels, for example, a valve in a vein or adjacent to the vessels. Ultrasound systems can also assist physicians because they can turn on color Doppler so that there is no doubt of whether the structure is a vein or artery.

Ultrasound-Guided Fine-Needle Aspiration or Biopsy

Ultrasound-guided fine-needle aspirations and biopsies are common exams done in an ultrasound laboratory. These studies use ultrasound to improve diagnostic confidence because physicians can actually track the needle going into the target tissue or fluid in question. The material that is removed can then be sent to the laboratory for further evaluation. Ultrasound also serves as an aid to avoid anatomical structures such as blood vessel and nerves as the needle is being inserted. It is important that the region of interest is scanned and shown to the clinician performing the procedure. The sonographer should be sure that all consent forms and supplies are present and to maintain a sterile field. It is important that the physician has the correct supplies so that once the material is withdrawn, it can quickly be sent to the laboratory for further evaluation. Common fine-needle aspiration procedures include thyroid or parathyroid nodules, lymph nodes, breast cysts, or superficial abscesses. Biopsies may include tissue from the breast, prostate, and liver.

Role of Sonographer

Sonographers are often required to assist during needle biopsy procedures. The sonographer must make sure to have the correct patient and explain the procedure to him or her before the clinician comes into the room. Any prior imaging exam and report should be provided for the physician. It is important that all consent forms are in the room so that the patient can sign them (either on paper or electronically) after they speak with the physician that will be performing the procedure. The sonographer will set up the sterile tray and gather any necessary supplies that the clinician may need. It is important to maintain a sterile field during the procedure to prevent an infection. The sonographer will often be scanning during the procedure, so communication with the physician is crucial in order to reach the target and save the necessary images so that the radiologist can generate a report. The patient should closely monitor the patient during the procedure, wipe off any gel, and provide follow-up information after the procedure including how the patient will receive their results. Sonographers should be sure that the collection containers are sent to the laboratory as soon as possible with the correct patient identifiers.

Assistance and Guidance of Sonographers During Procedures

Sonographers offer various types of assistance during ultrasound procedures. Regardless of the type of exam, the patient's safety is the most important concern of the sonographer. If a physician will be performing an ultrasound-guided procedure, the sonographer will have many roles. The sonographer must make sure that the correct patient, exam, and consent forms are gathered along with prior exams and reports. Sterile trays should be set up with other necessary supplies available. The sonographer should choose the correct equipment and ultrasound settings in order to obtain optimal resolution. It is important that enough space is available for the physician and that he or she can easily access the patient as well as see the ultrasound monitor. If the sonographer is to scan the patient, it is imperative to don sterile gloves and practice aseptic technique. If any specimens are collected, it is important that the sonographer correctly identifies them and sends them to the laboratory as soon as possible. Postprocedural steps include watching for signs of infection or bleeding and indicating how the patient will receive results.

Ultrasound Guidance for Injections

In the past, if physicians used guidance to inject a patient, it was often done by fluoroscopy; which is live X-ray. X-rays obviously use ionizing radiation, and the equipment is large and expensive. Ultrasound has become a more common method for physicians wanting a low-cost, nonionizing, portable technique for injections. Ultrasound-guided joint injections are performed to aid the physician when injecting corticosteroids that are used to help relieve pain and inflammation. Hyaluronic acid can be injected into the knee joint to provide a cushion and lubricate the knee joint to remove some of the pain from osteoarthritis. Ultrasound can be used to make sure the needle is in the correct location to provide the optimum amount of relief to the patient instead of having the physician inject blindly. Ultrasound also gives extra information to the physician so that other anatomical structures such as blood vessels and nerves can be avoided during an injection.

ARDMS Practice Test

Want to take this practice test in an online interactive format?
Check out the online resources page, which includes interactive practice questions and much more:
mometrix.com/resources719/ardmsabd

1. Caroli's disease may be characterized as which of the following?

a. Gallbladder wall thickening
b. Pneumobilia
c. Multiple cystic structures in the liver that communicate with the biliary tree
d. Dilation of the intrahepatic ducts with hydropic gallbladder

2. The "wheel within a wheel" sign is associated with which of the following pathologies?

a. Echinococcal cyst
b. Schistosomiasis
c. Liver metastases
d. Candidiasis

3. All of the following abdominal anatomic structures are retroperitoneal except the:

a. liver.
b. kidney.
c. aorta.
d. inferior vena cava.

4. What is the most common renal malignancy seen among adults?

a. Transitional cell carcinoma
b. Wilms' tumor
c. Cholangiocarcinoma
d. Renal cell carcinoma

5. The layers of the gallbladder, in the order of outer to inner layers, are:

a. serosal, muscular, subserous, epithelial mucosal.
b. epithelial mucosal, subserous, muscular, serosal.
c. serosal, subserous, epithelial mucosal, muscular.
d. serosal, subserous, muscular, epithelial mucosal.

6. The ______ duct drains the gallbladder and forms the common bile duct.

a. cystic
b. common hepatic
c. right hepatic
d. left hepatic

7. The following statement is false regarding the hormone cholecystokinin.

a. It promotes the release of bile from the gallbladder.
b. It aides in digestion.
c. It is stimulated by the smell of food.
d. It is released into the bloodstream.

8. Which vessel is routed posterior to the inferior vena cava?

a. Splenic artery
b. Right renal artery
c. Left renal artery
d. Superior mesenteric artery

9. In order to rule out choledocholithiasis, the sonographer would look for the presence of:

a. stones within the common bile duct.
b. a contracted gallbladder.
c. WES sign.
d. Murphy's sign.

10. Universal precautions that should be taken prior to, during, and after an ultrasound exam include all of the following except:

a. washing hands between patients.
b. using gloves and gowns when necessary.
c. disposing of blood-covered materials into the trash.
d. covering probes with sterile covers when necessary.

11. The patient may be instructed to move into all of the following positions to evaluate the gallbladder except:

a. erect.
b. right lateral decubitus.
c. left lateral decubitus.
d. supine.

12. Which transducer will provide superior imaging of a pediatric abdominal ultrasound?

a. 8 MHz curved array
b. 1 MHz linear array
c. 5 MHz curved array
d. 5 MHz sector

13. A renal sonogram is performed on a 67-year-old male. The sonographic findings are consistent with what appears to be a large, anechoic cyst in the upper pole of the left kidney. Increased brightness is visualized posterior to the anechoic area. Which type of sonographic artifact, when demonstrated, may best illustrate the diagnosis?

a. Shadowing
b. Ring down
c. Enhancement
d. Aliasing

14. Evaluation of the main portal vein with spectral Doppler analysis demonstrates all of the following except:

a. hepatofugal flow.
b. hepatopetal flow.
c. above the base line waveform.
d. red color of the MPV.

15. Multiple cysts ranging in size are visualized within the right kidney. The left kidney does not demonstrate any renal cysts. What is the most likely diagnosis?

a. Adult polycystic disease
b. Multicystic dysplasia
c. Childhood polycystic disease
d. Hydronephrosis

16. Evaluation of which structure is best visualized with a high-frequency transducer?

a. Proximal abdominal aorta
b. A palpable lump on the dorsal wrist
c. Mid-common carotid artery
d. Distal superficial femoral vein

17. Pertinent information that must be obtained prior to performing a fine needle aspiration of the thyroid includes all of the following except:

a. reviewing prior imaging and reports.
b. a signed and dated script for an FNA of the thyroid.
c. a signed consent form.
d. a prepared sterile tray.

18. The testicles are suspended within the scrotum by the:

a. vas deferens.
b. epididymis.
c. seminiferous tubules.
d. spermatic cord.

19. The least invasive type of thyroid biopsy that may be performed on a solitary thyroid nodule is a(n):

a. fine needle aspiration.
b. complete thyroidectomy.
c. core biopsy.
d. excisional biopsy.

20. A 16-year-old male presents to the emergency department with left-sided scrotal pain, nausea, and vomiting for the past several hours. He denies any recent trauma to his genitals. During sonographic evaluation, an enlarged left testicle with decreased echogenicity was documented. After further evaluation with color and spectral Doppler, intratesticular vasculature was noted to be absent. The patient most likely presents with:

a. orchitis.
b. torsion.
c. an abscess.
d. a hematocele.

21. Which arteries course along the renal pyramids within the kidney?

a. Segmental arteries
b. Arcuate arteries
c. Interlobular arteries
d. Interlobar arteries

22. A 27-year-old female presents to the ultrasound department for evaluation of the spleen. The patient complains of left upper quadrant pain. She was in a motor vehicle accident that occurred six months ago. All of the following sonographic findings may be present except:

a. hypovolemic shock.
b. left pleural effusion.
c. splenomegaly.
d. hematoma.

23. The portal triad includes the:

a. common bile duct, common hepatic duct, and the main portal vein.
b. common bile duct, hepatic vein, and the main portal vein.
c. common hepatic duct, hepatic artery, and the main portal vein.
d. common bile duct, hepatic artery, and the main portal vein.

24. Twinkling artifact may aid in the diagnosis of:

a. cholelithiasis.
b. hemangioma.
c. portal hypertension.
d. abdominal aortic aneurysm.

25. A 68-year-old male presents to the ultrasound department for evaluation of the liver. The patient complains of having anorexia, fatigue, and weakness for the past several months. His abdomen is enlarged. His labs indicate an increase in serum alpha-fetoprotein. Which is the most likely diagnosis?

a. Focal nodular hyperplasia
b. Hepatoma
c. Cavernous hemangioma
d. Liver cell adenoma

26. Which of the following is false regarding acute tubular necrosis?

a. It is the most common cause of renal failure
b. It causes an increase in arteriole resistance
c. It causes a decrease in arteriole resistance
d. It results in normal echogenicity of the renal cortex

27. The ureter inserts into the bladder at the trigone posteriorly and:

a. medially.
b. laterally.
c. superiorly.
d. inferiorly.

28. When acute pancreatitis is present, serum amylase and lipase levels both:

a. increase at the same rate, but lipase concentration stays elevated longer.
b. increase at the same rate, but amylase concentration stays elevated longer.
c. decrease at the same rate, but lipase concentration stays decreased longer.
d. decrease at the same rate, but amylase concentration stays decreased longer.

29. The main pancreatic duct is also known as the:

a. common bile duct.
b. duct of Santorini.
c. duct of Wirsung.
d. duct of Vater.

30. Clinical indications that may warrant a sonogram of the parathyroid gland to rule out a parathyroid adenoma include all of the following except:

a. hypophosphatemia.
b. hypercalcemia.
c. hypoparathyroidism.
d. hyperparathyroidism.

31. A patient presents to the ultrasound department for evaluation of the gallbladder. The patient complains of a recent onset of RUQ pain, nausea, and vomiting. The halo sign is visualized sonographically. What is the most likely diagnosis?

a. Acute cholecystitis
b. Chronic cholecystitis
c. Cholelithiasis
d. The patient has not been fasting

32. Which of the following indication may warrant a sonogram of the scrotum?

a. Trauma
b. Infertility
c. Scrotal enlargement
d. All of the above

33. Which of following vessels is NOT a branch of the celiac trunk?

a. Common hepatic artery
b. Right gastric artery
c. Left gastric artery
d. Splenic artery

34. A sonographic longitudinal image of the proximal aorta is obtained. Anteriorly, a vessel is visualized coursing inferiorly and parallel to the aorta. Which vessel is most likely being visualized?

a. Celiac trunk
b. Inferior mesenteric artery
c. Superior mesenteric artery
d. Left renal artery

35. The mediastinum of the testicle is a linear structure coursing within the testicle that appears sonographically as:

a. anechoic.
b. hypoechoic.
c. hyperechoic.
d. sonolucent.

36. The spleen is located within which of the following quadrants?

a. RUQ
b. RLQ
c. LUQ
d. LLQ

37. Sonographically, two anechoic structures are visualized within the head of the pancreas. Which structure is located in the anterior lateral portion of the pancreas head?

a. Distal common bile duct
b. Gastroduodenal artery
c. Splenic vein
d. Main pancreatic duct

38. A fold in the fundal portion of the gallbladder is most likely:

a. a junctional fold.
b. a Phrygian cap.
c. Hartman's pouch.
d. a subtotal division.

39. A contracted gallbladder may demonstrate the WES sign sonographically. What does WES stand for?

a. Wall edge stone
b. Wall edge shadow
c. Wall echo stone
d. Wall echo shadow

40. A patient presents for an ultrasound evaluation of the gallbladder. The patient complains of RUQ pain, nausea, and vomiting for several weeks. A distended gallbladder with thin walls is visualized. Based on the given information, what is the most likely diagnosis?

a. Acalculous cholecystitis
b. Acute calculous cholecystitis
c. Hydropic gallbladder
d. Chronic cholecystitis

41. A occlusion of the intrahepatic portal vein occurs, resulting in portal hypertension, which is visualized sonographically. What is the most likely diagnosis?

a. Schistosomiasis
b. Hepatitis
c. Cirrhosis
d. Fatty infiltration

42. Hepatomegaly is considered when the adult liver measures greater than:

a. 12cm.
b. 16cm.
c. 18cm.
d. 20cm.

43. Medullary nephrocalcinosis may present with all of the following except:

a. hyperparathyroidism.
b. hypercalcuria.
c. hypercalcemia.
d. hypocalcemia.

44. The sonographic findings associated with portal hypertension may include all the following except:

a. dilated portal veins.
b. development of collaterals.
c. hypoechoic liver parenchyma.
d. splenomegaly.

45. A 28-year-old female presents to the ultrasound department for an evaluation of the liver. The patient complains of RUQ pain and admits to a long history of oral contraceptive use. Several homogenous, well-defined, hyperechoic masses are visualized. What is the most likely diagnosis?

a. Adenoma
b. Cavernous hemangioma
c. Abscess
d. Hepatoblastoma

46. Which of the following would be a sonographic finding associated with an islet cell tumor of the pancreas?

a. A poorly defined hypoechoic mass
b. A mass located within the pancreatic head
c. Calcifications
d. Ascites

47. A patient presents for an ultrasound evaluation of the spleen. The patient complains of fever, and has an enlarged spleen on physical examination. Sonographically, a target lesion is documented. What is the most likely diagnosis?

a. Hamartoma
b. Metastases
c. Cavernous lymphangioma
d. Splenic candidiasis

48. The area positioned halfway between the right iliac crest and the umbilicus is described as:

a. McBurney's point.
b. McBurney's sign.
c. the target point.
d. Morison's point.

49. What is the most common type of thyroid carcinoma?

a. Papillary
b. Follicular
c. Anaplastic
d. Medullary

50. A contracted, biconcave, hyperechoic gallbladder is demonstrated sonographically. What is the most likely diagnosis?

a. Hydropic gallbladder
b. Porcelain gallbladder
c. Courvoisier gallbladder
d. Gallbladder sludge

Answer Key and Explanations

1. C: Multiple cystic structures in the liver that communicate with the biliary tree

Caroli's disease is characterized sonographically as multiple cystic structures in the liver that communicate with the biliary tree. Dilated ducts may display stones or sludge within.

2. D: Candidiasis

Candidiasis is described as having a "wheel within a wheel," or a target appearance on the sonogram. Liver metastases may also demonstrate a target appearance, but they are characterized as a bull's eye. Echinococcal cysts have multiple appearances sonographically, which include the water lily sign, honeycomb sign, and mother/daughter cyst. Schistosomiasis affects the portal vein and causes hypertrophy of the left lobe of the liver.

3. A: Liver

The liver is an intraperitoneal organ. The other choices are all located in the retroperitoneal space.

4. D: Renal cell carcinoma

Renal cell carcinoma is the most common primary renal malignancy in adults. Transitional cell carcinoma accounts for the majority of tumors affecting the lining of the collecting system. Wilms' tumor is the most common malignant abdominal mass among children. Cholangiocarcinoma is a type of cancer that affects the bile ducts of the liver.

5. D: Serosal, subserous, muscular, epithelial mucosal

The layers of the gallbladder, in the order from outer to inner layers include serosal, subserous, muscular, and epithelial mucosal layers.

6. A: Cystic duct

The cystic duct drains bile from the gallbladder. The right and left hepatic ducts merge to form the common hepatic duct. The common hepatic duct merges with the cystic duct to form the common bile duct.

7. C: It is stimulated by the smell of food.

Cholecystokinin is a hormone that is released into the bloodstream when chyme enters the intestinal tract. In its presence, bile will be ejected into the cystic duct. The bile will travel to the common bile duct where it is ejected into the duodenum via the sphincter of Oddi, located at the head of the pancreas. In order for the hormone to be released into the bloodstream, chyme must be present in the duodenum, which would occur after eating, rather than simply smelling food.

8. B: Right renal artery

The right renal artery originates off the anterolateral aorta. It courses toward the right renal hilum, passing posterior to the inferior vena cava. The splenic artery and the superior mesenteric artery course anterior to aorta. The left renal artery courses toward the left renal hilum.

9. A: Stones within the common bile duct

The presence of stones within the common bile duct defines choledocholithiasis.

10. C: Disposing of blood-covered materials into the trash

Universal precautions involve avoiding contact with and disposing of bodily fluids safely. Hand washing, using gloves and gowns, and utilizing sterile covers are several precautions that may be taken to protect the technologist from these bodily fluids. Proper disposal of blood-covered materials includes the use of biohazard bags and bins. Nothing with blood should ever be thrown into the trash.

11. B: Right lateral decubitus

The standard protocol for the evaluation of the gallbladder involves the supine and left lateral decubitus positions. Having the patient sit erect or semi-erect may be appropriate when gallstones appear to be non-mobile. The right lateral decubitus position is more commonly used for the evaluation of the spleen, the left kidney, and sometimes the aorta.

12. A: 8 MHz curved array

An 8 MHz curved array transducer will provide the superior imaging of a pediatric abdomen compared to the other choices. The higher-frequency transducer provides a better resolution of the images. A pediatric abdomen will benefit from a higher-frequency probe because less penetration is needed due to smaller body size. Linear probes tend not to be used for abdominal ultrasounds; even though the frequency is higher, the probe type is not adequate. Sector transducers tend to be used for scanning through the rib spaces on difficult abdomens.

13. C: Enhancement

Enhancement artifact occurs when sound waves pass through a weakly attenuating structure, producing increased brightness posterior to the area. This artifact is beneficial when trying to determine if a renal mass is cystic or solid. Aliasing is a Doppler artifact that occurs when the Doppler shift exceeds the Nyquist limit. Shadowing is the opposite of enhancement. Ring down artifact occurs posterior to a reflector as parallel bands.

14. A: Hepatofugal flow

Hepatofugal flow is blood flow traveling away from the liver. The main portal vein is the main source of oxygenated blood to the liver. The flow is traveling toward the liver and is called hepatopetal flow. Since this vessel is carrying oxygenated blood toward the liver, spectral and Doppler evaluation will demonstrate a red vessel with flow above the baseline.

15. B: Multicystic dysplasia

Multicystic dysplasia is a unilateral disease that demonstrates multiple cysts of varying size in one kidney. Adult polycystic and childhood polycystic disease are both bilateral diseases. Hydronephrosis may appear as multiple parapelvic cysts which all stretch out and connect to the renal pelvis.

16. B: A palpable lump on the dorsal wrist

A high-frequency transducer will provide the best sonographic images of a palpable lump on the dorsal wrist. Higher-frequency transducers provide an image with a higher resolution, but lack penetration. Superficial tissues will be best evaluated with a higher-frequency probe. The other choices may be best evaluated with a lower-frequency probe due to their anatomic locations. They are located deeper in the body than a palpable lump.

17. D: A prepared sterile tray

Though a prepared sterile tray is necessary for a fine needle aspiration of the thyroid, it is not pertinent information. Reviewing prior images and reports, a script from the referring physician, and a signed consent form are all pertinent information that must be obtained prior to an invasive procedure such as an ultrasound-guided FNA of the thyroid.

18. D: Spermatic cord

The spermatic cord suspends the testicles in the scrotum. The vas deferens transports sperm to the urethra. The epididymis stores and excretes sperm. The seminiferous tubules produce sperm.

19. A: Fine needle aspiration

A fine needle aspiration (FNA) of the thyroid gland is a minimally-invasive procedure that involves the use of a very thin needle, usually an 18 to 25-gauge needle. The needle is guided directly into the nodule under ultrasound and is moved around within the nodule to shear off as many cells as possible. An FNA is the least invasive of the procedures listed, but warrants the poorest results. An excisional biopsy or a complete thyroidectomy are more invasive but allow the pathologist to examine the tissue makeup, which increases the chance of a definite diagnosis. A core biopsy also provides the pathologist with a larger sample of tissue. An FNA provides the pathologist with cells examined under cytology, whereas the other choices provide the pathologist with tissue samples examined under histology and increase the chance of diagnosis.

20. B: Torsion

Torsion occurs when the spermatic cord becomes twisted, cutting off blood supply to the testicle. It occurs more commonly in adolescents than in adults and more often in the left testicle. The patient may present with scrotal pain, nausea, and vomiting. Sonographically, the testicle may appear enlarged with decreased echogenicity, a hydrocele may be present, and interrogation of the intratesticular vasculature may be absent with color and power Doppler evaluation. Torsion is considered a medical emergency and must be treated immediately to prevent complete infarction of the testicle. Orchitis is inflammation of the testes and presents as scrotal pain. Sonographically, orchitis may have a variable appearance ranging from hypoechoic with hyperemic vasculature under color and spectral Doppler evaluation to atrophic testes. Abscess may occur due to untreated orchitis. The patient may present with scrotal pain and swelling. An avascular, sonolucent, or complex mass may be seen on the sonogram. A hematocele most often occurs after trauma and causes blood to accumulate within the scrotum. It often mimics torsion and varies in sonographic appearances from sonolucent to complex with septations.

21. D: Interlobar arteries

The main renal artery enters the renal hilum and branches into the segmental arteries. The segmental arteries then course through the renal pelvis region and branch into the interlobar arteries. These arteries course along the renal pyramids, pass over the base of the pyramids, and branch into the arcuate arteries. The arcuate arteries branch into the interlobular arteries.

22. A: Hypovolemic shock

Hypovolemic shock is caused by severe blood loss and may result in multiple organ failure. The patient may present with systemic symptoms of hypovolemic shock; therefore, it is not a sonographic appearance of the spleen. Left pleural effusion, splenomegaly, and a hematoma are pathologies that will be displayed sonographically.

23. D: Common bile duct, hepatic artery, and the main portal vein

The common bile duct, hepatic artery, and the main portal vein make up the portal triad. Sonographically, the "Mickey Mouse" sign may be visualized at the porta hepatis. The hepatic vein contains the right, left, and middle branches, which converge with the inferior vena cava. The common hepatic duct converges with the cystic duct to form the common bile duct. The hepatic duct and the hepatic vein are not part of the portal triad.

24. A: Cholelithiasis

Twinkling artifact aids in the diagnosis of gallstones. When color Doppler is applied, a twinkle of color is visualized posterior to the stone where shadowing would be displayed. A hemangioma may show enhancement artifact. Portal hypertension and an abdominal aortic aneurysm will not display twinkling artifact.

25. B: Hepatoma

Hepatoma (hepatocellular carcinoma) is the most common primary liver malignancy. Patients may present with hepatomegaly; and elevated levels of AST, ALT, and serum AFP. Focal nodular hyperplasia, cavernous hemangioma, and liver cell adenoma are all benign neoplasms of the liver. They may show similar signs and symptoms, or they may be asymptomatic.

26. C: It causes a decrease in arteriole resistance

Acute tubular necrosis is the most common cause of renal failure. Renal failure occurs due to ischemia, causing an increase in arteriole resistance. The echogenicity in the majority of cases does not change from its normal sonographic appearance.

27. D: Inferiorly

The ureter inserts into the trigone posteriorly and inferiorly.

28. A: Increase at the same rate, but lipase concentration stays elevated longer

In the presence of acute pancreatitis, serum amylase and lipase increase at the same rate but lipase will stay elevated longer than amylase.

29. C: Duct of Wirsung

The duct of Wirsung is the main pancreatic duct that joins the common bile duct within the pancreatic head at the Ampulla of Vater where they dump into the second portion of the duodenum. The duct of Santorini is the accessory duct of the pancreas.

30. C: Hypoparathyroidism

Hypophosphatemia, hypercalcemia, and hyperparathyroidism are all clinical indications that would warrant a sonogram to rule out a parathyroid adenoma.

31. A: Acute cholecystitis

Acute cholecystitis can be characterized by the halo sign sonographically. The halo sign describes a thick, edematous gallbladder wall. A non-fasting patient may also demonstrate a similar appearance, which is why it is important to take a good patient history. Chronic cholecystitis is visualized as a contracted gallbladder with thick, hyperechoic walls. Cholelithiasis is characterized as gallstones.

32. D: All of the above

Ultrasound evaluation of the scrotum may be indicated for trauma, infertility, or scrotal enlargement.

33. B: Right gastric artery

The common hepatic artery branches off the celiac trunk and courses toward the porta hepatis. The left gastric artery branches off the celiac trunk and courses toward the stomach. It is not typically visualized sonographically. The splenic artery branches off the celiac trunk and courses toward the splenic hilum. This vessel tends to be tortuous. Only the right gastric artery is not part of the celiac trunk.

34. C: Superior mesenteric artery

The superior mesenteric artery is the second branch of the aorta. It branches anteriorly off the aorta and travels distally and parallel to the aorta, supplying portions of the small and large intestine. The celiac trunk is the first branch of the aorta. It branches anteriorly and trifurcates into the left gastric artery, common hepatic artery, and the splenic artery. The longitudinal view of the renal arteries is best visualized in the transverse scanning plane. The inferior mesenteric artery branches off the aorta near the aortic bifurcation.

35. C: Hyperechoic

The mediastinum is visualized sonographically as a hyperechoic linear structure.

36. C: LUQ

The spleen is located within the left upper quadrant. It is found specifically within the left hypochondriac region, with the superior portion extending into the epigastric region.

37. B: Gastroduodenal artery

The gastroduodenal artery is located in the anterior and lateral portion of the pancreatic head. The common bile duct is located in the posterolateral portion of the pancreatic head. The splenic vein is located posterior to the pancreas and converges with the superior mesenteric vein and the inferior mesenteric vein to form the main portal vein. The main pancreatic duct may be visualized within the body of the pancreas but is not usually seen sonographically.

38. B: Phrygian cap

A Phrygian cap is a fold of the fundal portion of the gallbladder. A junctional fold is seen between the body and the neck of the gallbladder. It is the most common variant. A Hartman's pouch is the curvy neck of the gallbladder. Subtotal division of the gallbladder appears as two lumens with only one cystic duct.

39. D: Wall echo shadow

Wall echo shadow is the correct meaning of the abbreviation of the WES sign.

40. C: Hydropic gallbladder

Hydropic gallbladder is distention of the gallbladder without the presence of gallbladder wall thickening. Acute calculous cholecystitis will demonstrate gallstones and gallbladder wall thickening. The patient may present with similar symptoms. Acalculous cholecystitis is visualized as a thickened gallbladder wall without the presence of gallstones. Chronic cholecystitis may appear as a fibrotic gallbladder wall along with a contracted gallbladder.

41. A: Schistosomiasis

Schistosomiasis is an infection that occurs when a parasite enters the body and travels to the lung or liver. Sonographic evaluation may demonstrate increased echogenicity of the portal walls or thickened portal walls, and portosystemic collaterals may be visualized. Hepatitis may demonstrate prominent portal vein walls, but no occlusion. Cirrhosis and fatty infiltration may make it difficult to visualize the portal vein walls. Fatty infiltration causes increased echogenicity of the liver parenchyma, making evaluation of the portal veins difficult. Cirrhosis also causes increased attenuation of the liver parenchyma, causing poor visualization of the portal vein margins.

42. B: 16cm

The AP dimension of the liver is considered enlarged when it measures greater than 16cm.

43. D: Hypocalcemia

Hypocalcemia is a decrease of calcium in the blood. Medullary nephrocalcinosis is the buildup of calcium in the distal convoluted tubules and the loops of Henle.

44. C: Hypoechoic liver parenchyma

The liver parenchyma associated with portal hypertension tends to be hyperechoic due to increased attenuation. Portal hypertension is a result of an underlying pathology such as infection. The liver parenchyma, when inflamed from infection, will result in a hyperechoic appearance sonographically. Dilated portal veins, the development of collaterals, and enlargement of the spleen or liver have all been associated with portal hypertension.

45. B: Cavernous hemangioma

A cavernous hemangioma is the most common benign liver mass. It may be caused by the extended use of oral contraceptives and it is more prevalent in women. Sonographically, a hemangioma may appear as a homogenous, well-defined, hyperechoic mass. An adenoma tends to display as a solid or a hypoechoic mass. An abscess is visualized as a complex mass and may display acoustic enhancement. A hepatoblastoma may appear as a heterogeneous hyperechoic mass or as a complex mass with internal septations.

46. C: Calcifications

Sonographically, an Islet cell tumor of the pancreas may be displayed as a well-defined hypoechoic mass with calcifications or necrosis, and it tends to be located in the body or tail.

47. D: Splenic candidiasis

Splenic candidiasis presents clinically with splenomegaly and fever. Sonographically, it appears as a target lesion. A hamartoma, metastases, and cavernous lymphangioma are all asymptomatic. Metastases may appear similar sonographically but the patient is usually symptom free.

48. A: McBurney's point

McBurney's point is the area halfway between the right iliac crest and the umbilicus. This area is pressed on to rule out rebound pain that is associated with appendicitis.

49. A: Papillary

Papillary carcinoma is the most common type of thyroid carcinoma. Follicular carcinoma is the second most common, and anaplastic and medullary types are less common.

50. B: Porcelain gallbladder

A porcelain gallbladder is described as a completely calcified gallbladder wall. Sonographically, it may display as a contracted, biconcave, hyperechoic gallbladder. Hydropic gallbladder is an enlarged gallbladder usually exceeding five centimeters in diameter. Courvoisier gallbladder demonstrates gallbladder distention greater than four centimeters in diameter. Gallbladder sludge is low-amplitude echoes layering in the dependant portion of the gallbladder.

How to Overcome Test Anxiety

Just the thought of taking a test is enough to make most people a little nervous. A test is an important event that can have a long-term impact on your future, so it's important to take it seriously and it's natural to feel anxious about performing well. But just because anxiety is normal, that doesn't mean that it's helpful in test taking, or that you should simply accept it as part of your life. Anxiety can have a variety of effects. These effects can be mild, like making you feel slightly nervous, or severe, like blocking your ability to focus or remember even a simple detail.

If you experience test anxiety—whether severe or mild—it's important to know how to beat it. To discover this, first you need to understand what causes test anxiety.

Causes of Test Anxiety

While we often think of anxiety as an uncontrollable emotional state, it can actually be caused by simple, practical things. One of the most common causes of test anxiety is that a person does not feel adequately prepared for their test. This feeling can be the result of many different issues such as poor study habits or lack of organization, but the most common culprit is time management. Starting to study too late, failing to organize your study time to cover all of the material, or being distracted while you study will mean that you're not well prepared for the test. This may lead to cramming the night before, which will cause you to be physically and mentally exhausted for the test. Poor time management also contributes to feelings of stress, fear, and hopelessness as you realize you are not well prepared but don't know what to do about it.

Other times, test anxiety is not related to your preparation for the test but comes from unresolved fear. This may be a past failure on a test, or poor performance on tests in general. It may come from comparing yourself to others who seem to be performing better or from the stress of living up to expectations. Anxiety may be driven by fears of the future—how failure on this test would affect your educational and career goals. These fears are often completely irrational, but they can still negatively impact your test performance.

Elements of Test Anxiety

As mentioned earlier, test anxiety is considered to be an emotional state, but it has physical and mental components as well. Sometimes you may not even realize that you are suffering from test anxiety until you notice the physical symptoms. These can include trembling hands, rapid heartbeat, sweating, nausea, and tense muscles. Extreme anxiety may lead to fainting or vomiting. Obviously, any of these symptoms can have a negative impact on testing. It is important to recognize them as soon as they begin to occur so that you can address the problem before it damages your performance.

The mental components of test anxiety include trouble focusing and inability to remember learned information. During a test, your mind is on high alert, which can help you recall information and stay focused for an extended period of time. However, anxiety interferes with your mind's natural processes, causing you to blank out, even on the questions you know well. The strain of testing during anxiety makes it difficult to stay focused, especially on a test that may take several hours. Extreme anxiety can take a huge mental toll, making it difficult not only to recall test information but even to understand the test questions or pull your thoughts together.

Effects of Test Anxiety

Test anxiety is like a disease—if left untreated, it will get progressively worse. Anxiety leads to poor performance, and this reinforces the feelings of fear and failure, which in turn lead to poor performances on subsequent tests. It can grow from a mild nervousness to a crippling condition. If allowed to progress, test anxiety can have a big impact on your schooling, and consequently on your future.

Test anxiety can spread to other parts of your life. Anxiety on tests can become anxiety in any stressful situation, and blanking on a test can turn into panicking in a job situation. But fortunately, you don't have to let anxiety rule your testing and determine your grades. There are a number of relatively simple steps you can take to move past anxiety and function normally on a test and in the rest of life.

Physical Steps for Beating Test Anxiety

While test anxiety is a serious problem, the good news is that it can be overcome. It doesn't have to control your ability to think and remember information. While it may take time, you can begin taking steps today to beat anxiety.

Just as your first hint that you may be struggling with anxiety comes from the physical symptoms, the first step to treating it is also physical. Rest is crucial for having a clear, strong mind. If you are tired, it is much easier to give in to anxiety. But if you establish good sleep habits, your body and mind will be ready to perform optimally, without the strain of exhaustion. Additionally, sleeping well helps you to retain information better, so you're more likely to recall the answers when you see the test questions.

Getting good sleep means more than going to bed on time. It's important to allow your brain time to relax. Take study breaks from time to time so it doesn't get overworked, and don't study right before bed. Take time to rest your mind before trying to rest your body, or you may find it difficult to fall asleep.

Along with sleep, other aspects of physical health are important in preparing for a test. Good nutrition is vital for good brain function. Sugary foods and drinks may give a burst of energy but this burst is followed by a crash, both physically and emotionally. Instead, fuel your body with protein and vitamin-rich foods.

Also, drink plenty of water. Dehydration can lead to headaches and exhaustion, especially if your brain is already under stress from the rigors of the test. Particularly if your test is a long one, drink water during the breaks. And if possible, take an energy-boosting snack to eat between sections.

Along with sleep and diet, a third important part of physical health is exercise. Maintaining a steady workout schedule is helpful, but even taking 5-minute study breaks to walk can help get your blood pumping faster and clear your head. Exercise also releases endorphins, which contribute to a positive feeling and can help combat test anxiety.

When you nurture your physical health, you are also contributing to your mental health. If your body is healthy, your mind is much more likely to be healthy as well. So take time to rest, nourish your body with healthy food and water, and get moving as much as possible. Taking these physical steps will make you stronger and more able to take the mental steps necessary to overcome test anxiety.

Mental Steps for Beating Test Anxiety

Working on the mental side of test anxiety can be more challenging, but as with the physical side, there are clear steps you can take to overcome it. As mentioned earlier, test anxiety often stems from lack of preparation, so the obvious solution is to prepare for the test. Effective studying may be the most important weapon you have for beating test anxiety, but you can and should employ several other mental tools to combat fear.

First, boost your confidence by reminding yourself of past success—tests or projects that you aced. If you're putting as much effort into preparing for this test as you did for those, there's no reason you should expect to fail here. Work hard to prepare; then trust your preparation.

Second, surround yourself with encouraging people. It can be helpful to find a study group, but be sure that the people you're around will encourage a positive attitude. If you spend time with others who are anxious or cynical, this will only contribute to your own anxiety. Look for others who are motivated to study hard from a desire to succeed, not from a fear of failure.

Third, reward yourself. A test is physically and mentally tiring, even without anxiety, and it can be helpful to have something to look forward to. Plan an activity following the test, regardless of the outcome, such as going to a movie or getting ice cream.

When you are taking the test, if you find yourself beginning to feel anxious, remind yourself that you know the material. Visualize successfully completing the test. Then take a few deep, relaxing breaths and return to it. Work through the questions carefully but with confidence, knowing that you are capable of succeeding.

Developing a healthy mental approach to test taking will also aid in other areas of life. Test anxiety affects more than just the actual test—it can be damaging to your mental health and even contribute to depression. It's important to beat test anxiety before it becomes a problem for more than testing.

Study Strategy

Being prepared for the test is necessary to combat anxiety, but what does being prepared look like? You may study for hours on end and still not feel prepared. What you need is a strategy for test prep. The next few pages outline our recommended steps to help you plan out and conquer the challenge of preparation.

Step 1: Scope Out the Test

Learn everything you can about the format (multiple choice, essay, etc.) and what will be on the test. Gather any study materials, course outlines, or sample exams that may be available. Not only will this help you to prepare, but knowing what to expect can help to alleviate test anxiety.

Step 2: Map Out the Material

Look through the textbook or study guide and make note of how many chapters or sections it has. Then divide these over the time you have. For example, if a book has 15 chapters and you have five days to study, you need to cover three chapters each day. Even better, if you have the time, leave an extra day at the end for overall review after you have gone through the material in depth.

If time is limited, you may need to prioritize the material. Look through it and make note of which sections you think you already have a good grasp on, and which need review. While you are studying, skim quickly through the familiar sections and take more time on the challenging parts. Write out your plan so you don't get lost as you go. Having a written plan also helps you feel more in control of the study, so anxiety is less likely to arise from feeling overwhelmed at the amount to cover.

Step 3: Gather Your Tools

Decide what study method works best for you. Do you prefer to highlight in the book as you study and then go back over the highlighted portions? Or do you type out notes of the important information? Or is it helpful to make flashcards that you can carry with you? Assemble the pens, index cards, highlighters, post-it notes, and any other materials you may need so you won't be distracted by getting up to find things while you study.

If you're having a hard time retaining the information or organizing your notes, experiment with different methods. For example, try color-coding by subject with colored pens, highlighters, or post-it notes. If you learn better by hearing, try recording yourself reading your notes so you can listen while in the car, working out, or simply sitting at your desk. Ask a friend to quiz you from your flashcards, or try teaching someone the material to solidify it in your mind.

Step 4: Create Your Environment

It's important to avoid distractions while you study. This includes both the obvious distractions like visitors and the subtle distractions like an uncomfortable chair (or a too-comfortable couch that makes you want to fall asleep). Set up the best study environment possible: good lighting and a comfortable work area. If background music helps you focus, you may want to turn it on, but otherwise keep the room quiet. If you are using a computer to take notes, be sure you don't have any other windows open, especially applications like social media, games, or anything else that could distract you. Silence your phone and turn off notifications. Be sure to keep water close by so you stay hydrated while you study (but avoid unhealthy drinks and snacks).

Also, take into account the best time of day to study. Are you freshest first thing in the morning? Try to set aside some time then to work through the material. Is your mind clearer in the afternoon or evening? Schedule your study session then. Another method is to study at the same time of day that you will take the test, so that your brain gets used to working on the material at that time and will be ready to focus at test time.

Step 5: Study!

Once you have done all the study preparation, it's time to settle into the actual studying. Sit down, take a few moments to settle your mind so you can focus, and begin to follow your study plan. Don't give in to distractions or let yourself procrastinate. This is your time to prepare so you'll be ready to fearlessly approach the test. Make the most of the time and stay focused.

Of course, you don't want to burn out. If you study too long you may find that you're not retaining the information very well. Take regular study breaks. For example, taking five minutes out of every hour to walk briskly, breathing deeply and swinging your arms, can help your mind stay fresh.

As you get to the end of each chapter or section, it's a good idea to do a quick review. Remind yourself of what you learned and work on any difficult parts. When you feel that you've mastered the material, move on to the next part. At the end of your study session, briefly skim through your notes again.

But while review is helpful, cramming last minute is NOT. If at all possible, work ahead so that you won't need to fit all your study into the last day. Cramming overloads your brain with more information than it can process and retain, and your tired mind may struggle to recall even previously learned information when it is overwhelmed with last-minute study. Also, the urgent nature of cramming and the stress placed on your brain contribute to anxiety. You'll be more likely to go to the test feeling unprepared and having trouble thinking clearly.

So don't cram, and don't stay up late before the test, even just to review your notes at a leisurely pace. Your brain needs rest more than it needs to go over the information again. In fact, plan to finish your studies by noon or early afternoon the day before the test. Give your brain the rest of the day to relax or focus on other things, and get a good night's sleep. Then you will be fresh for the test and better able to recall what you've studied.

Step 6: Take a Practice Test

Many courses offer sample tests, either online or in the study materials. This is an excellent resource to check whether you have mastered the material, as well as to prepare for the test format and environment.

Check the test format ahead of time: the number of questions, the type (multiple choice, free response, etc.), and the time limit. Then create a plan for working through them. For example, if you have 30 minutes to take a 60-question test, your limit is 30 seconds per question. Spend less time on the questions you know well so that you can take more time on the difficult ones.

If you have time to take several practice tests, take the first one open book, with no time limit. Work through the questions at your own pace and make sure you fully understand them. Gradually work up to taking a test under test conditions: sit at a desk with all study materials put away and set a timer. Pace yourself to make sure you finish the test with time to spare and go back to check your answers if you have time.

After each test, check your answers. On the questions you missed, be sure you understand why you missed them. Did you misread the question (tests can use tricky wording)? Did you forget the information? Or was it something you hadn't learned? Go back and study any shaky areas that the practice tests reveal.

Taking these tests not only helps with your grade, but also aids in combating test anxiety. If you're already used to the test conditions, you're less likely to worry about it, and working through tests until you're scoring well gives you a confidence boost. Go through the practice tests until you feel comfortable, and then you can go into the test knowing that you're ready for it.

Test Tips

On test day, you should be confident, knowing that you've prepared well and are ready to answer the questions. But aside from preparation, there are several test day strategies you can employ to maximize your performance.

First, as stated before, get a good night's sleep the night before the test (and for several nights before that, if possible). Go into the test with a fresh, alert mind rather than staying up late to study.

Try not to change too much about your normal routine on the day of the test. It's important to eat a nutritious breakfast, but if you normally don't eat breakfast at all, consider eating just a protein bar. If you're a coffee drinker, go ahead and have your normal coffee. Just make sure you time it so that the caffeine doesn't wear off right in the middle of your test. Avoid sugary beverages, and drink enough water to stay hydrated but not so much that you need a restroom break 10 minutes into the test. If your test isn't first thing in the morning, consider going for a walk or doing a light workout before the test to get your blood flowing.

Allow yourself enough time to get ready, and leave for the test with plenty of time to spare so you won't have the anxiety of scrambling to arrive in time. Another reason to be early is to select a good seat. It's helpful to sit away from doors and windows, which can be distracting. Find a good seat, get out your supplies, and settle your mind before the test begins.

When the test begins, start by going over the instructions carefully, even if you already know what to expect. Make sure you avoid any careless mistakes by following the directions.

Then begin working through the questions, pacing yourself as you've practiced. If you're not sure on an answer, don't spend too much time on it, and don't let it shake your confidence. Either skip it and come back later, or eliminate as many wrong answers as possible and guess among the remaining ones. Don't dwell on these questions as you continue—put them out of your mind and focus on what lies ahead.

Be sure to read all of the answer choices, even if you're sure the first one is the right answer. Sometimes you'll find a better one if you keep reading. But don't second-guess yourself if you do immediately know the answer. Your gut instinct is usually right. Don't let test anxiety rob you of the information you know.

If you have time at the end of the test (and if the test format allows), go back and review your answers. Be cautious about changing any, since your first instinct tends to be correct, but make sure you didn't misread any of the questions or accidentally mark the wrong answer choice. Look over any you skipped and make an educated guess.

At the end, leave the test feeling confident. You've done your best, so don't waste time worrying about your performance or wishing you could change anything. Instead, celebrate the successful completion of this test. And finally, use this test to learn how to deal with anxiety even better next time.

Review Video: Test Anxiety
Visit mometrix.com/academy and enter code: 100340

Important Qualification

Not all anxiety is created equal. If your test anxiety is causing major issues in your life beyond the classroom or testing center, or if you are experiencing troubling physical symptoms related to your anxiety, it may be a sign of a serious physiological or psychological condition. If this sounds like your situation, we strongly encourage you to seek professional help.

Online Resources

Due to our efforts to try to keep this book to a manageable length, we've created a link that will give you access to all of your online resources:

mometrix.com/resources719/ardmsabd

It's Your Moment, Let's Celebrate It!

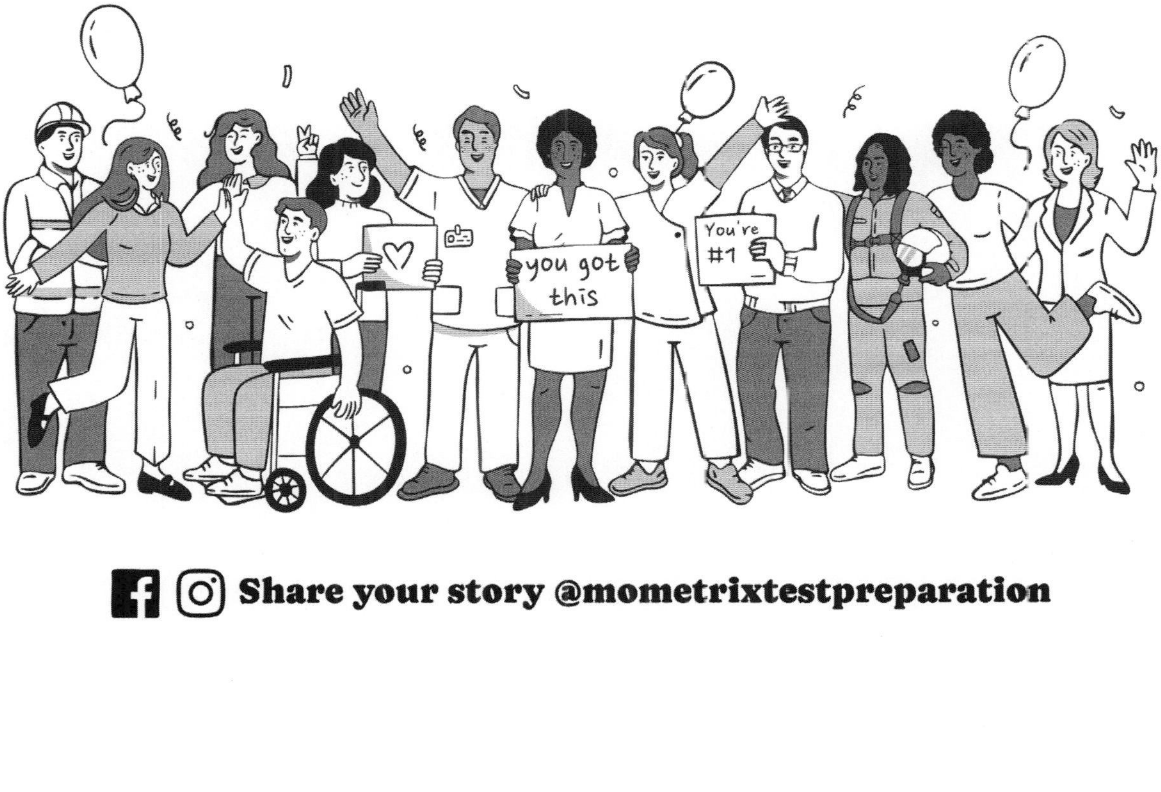

Share your story @mometrixtestpreparation